"Are you not aware that your body is a temple of the Holy Spirit in you, which you have from God, and you are not your own? For you are bought with a price. By all means glorify God in your body."

(1 Corinthians 6:19-20)

Your Personal Roadmap

to **Whole Body Cleansing**

Barbara Brown, MSE

Dr. Tom Taylor

"I pray that in all respects you may prosper and be in good health, just as your soul prospers." (3 John 2, NASB)

Your Personal Roadmap
to **Whole Body Cleansing**

Manufactured in the United States of America

ISBN: 978-1-929921-48-5 (PREMIUM EDITION – Color)
978-1-929921-18-8 (Regular Edition – B&W)
978-1-929921-35-5 (E-Pub)

Published by

Whole Life Whole Health, LLC. • Lake Dallas, TX 75065

The information contained in this book is based upon the research and personal and professional experience of the authors and other health care professionals who contributed to this body of knowledge. It is not intended to diagnose or treat any illness, or as a substitute for consulting with your health care provider.

Dedication

To the Father of us all:

May we take as much care of our bodies — these "earth suits" — as You did in making them in Your image.

You have provided everything we need to be healthy in spirit, soul and body. Thank You for the journey You've taken us through, in our quest for health and well-being. May our lives bring You honor and glory as we follow the path You've laid before us in Your word.

~~~~~~

Our thanks to the health care professionals and others whose input added richly to the body of knowledge contained here.

Our thanks also to the individuals and families who crossed our path looking for solutions with open minds and willing hearts. Their experiences and successes added immeasurably to our journey. We pray that millions more will be blessed!

"God put a piece of Himself into every cell of our bodies."

Barbara Brown, MSE
~~~~~~

Foreword

We have found the following principles to be 100 percent reliable:

SPIRITUAL PRINCIPLES

1. **Merging science and scripture is essential to gain clear understanding of how your body works, how you get sick, how you get healthy, and how you stay that way.**
2. **Scriptural principles are entirely practical, 100 percent reliable, and applicable, whether you believe them or not.**
3. **You are a spiritual being undergoing a physical experience, not the other way around. When you live like a physical being looking for a spiritual experience, you are 180 degrees out of phase with how God created you.**
4. **Pain, illness, disease, or dysfunction, is the inevitable result of being out of alignment with God's original blueprint.**
5. **Healing is also inevitable and unstoppable, when you align and agree with God's divine design.**

PHYSICAL PRINCIPLES

1. **Your body is self-organizing, self-healing, and self-regulating.**
2. **Your body does not think, judge or reason.**
3. **Your body responds for only one purpose, survival, and the response is perfect for the stimulus that makes it necessary.**
4. **Your body's responses don't always feel good (we call those symptoms), but they are perfect nevertheless.**

5. **Your body is an alkaline organism by design. It creates acid as a byproduct of being alive, and you add to that acid load by the choices you make in eight key areas** ***(see page 102)*****.**
6. **Your physical design (your anatomy) – tooth structure, digestive tract, enzyme production, and absorption process – is suited to a primarily plant-based diet.**
7. **Your body is constantly cleansing, rebuilding and supporting the life within every cell and between all cells.**

Principles like those above hold true no matter what your gender, race, ethnicity, or beliefs. The good news is that you are in charge of the choices that enable your body to perform at peak efficiency, according to its original design. Any level of performance less than that is the natural consequence of your choices in eight key areas discussed on page 102.

Finally, your body responds according to its design, not to your desire. You probably know people who genuinely want to be well, yet vibrant health seems to evade them. All our combined experience has proven that when you align yourself with God's design – spiritually, mentally, and physically – illness cannot hold you hostage; instead, health, happiness and success is the inevitable outcome.

Sound good?

Let's get on with it, shall we?

Barbara Brown, MSE

Dr. Tom Taylor

In the Beginning...

Then God said, "Let the land produce vegetation, seed-bearing plants and trees...that bear fruit with seed in it, according to their various kinds" and it was so...and God saw that it was good...Then God said, "I give you every seed-bearing plant on the face of the whole earth and every tree that has fruit in it. They will be yours for food." (Genesis 1:11-12, 29)

"Everything that lives and moves about will be food for you. Just as I gave you the green plants, I now give you everything..." (Genesis 9:3)

He waters the mountains from His upper chambers; the land is satisfied by the fruit of his work. He makes grass grow for the cattle, and plants for people to cultivate – bringing forth food from the earth: wine that gladdens human hearts, oil to make their faces shine, and bread that sustains their hearts. (Psalm 104:13-15)

"Take wheat and barley, beans and lentils, millet and spelt; put them in a storage jar and use them to make bread for yourself." (Ezekiel 4:9)

"Fruit trees of all kinds will grow on both banks of the river. Their leaves will not wither, nor will their fruit fail. Every month they will bear fruit, because the water from the sanctuary flows to them. Their fruit will serve for food and their leaves for healing."

(Ezekiel 47:12)

Daniel then said to the guard, *"Please test your servants for ten days: Give us nothing but vegetables to eat and water to drink."* At the end of ten days they looked healthier and better nourished than any of the young men who ate the royal food. (Daniel 1:11-12, 15)

Table of Contents

"Imagine how you'd look and smell if you never took a shower."

"If you've never gone through a cleanse, that's how you look and smell on the inside!"

"We are free to make our choices, but we are not free from the consequences of those choices."

Barbara Brown, MSE

Introduction

The word "cleanse" means to rid, free or purify. The term is not limited to the physical body; it also includes the soul and spirit. Many books have been written about cleansing, but unlike other books, we go beyond cleansing only the physical body.

The truth is, you are a spiritual being first, undergoing a physical experience. Your physical body is simply "along for the ride." This book is the result of decades of experience with thousands of doctor/patient/client encounters and is intended to be a "manual" for cleansing the soul and spirit, along with its "house."

Cleansing is critical to achieve health and wellness, but we have also provided the simplest, least expensive, and most reliable ways we've found to evaluate and monitor your *total* health and well-being.

We pray that you will enjoy the benefits of a clean body, soul and spirit!

Blessings on your journey,

Barbara Brown, MSE
Dr. Tom Taylor

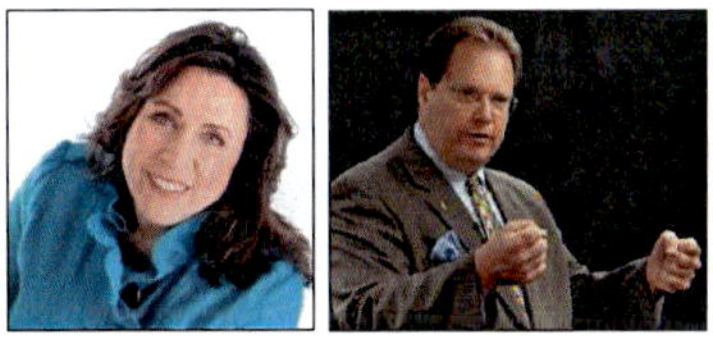

RESOURCES

"What do *you* do to stay young and healthy?" That's probably the most frequently asked question we hear. Here's the answer:

We do **five things** every day, no matter what, and so does every client we serve, because we're serious about keeping our bodies humming, having iron-clad immune systems and memories like steel traps, sleeping like babies, and otherwise living well in spirit, soul, and body.

Here they are:

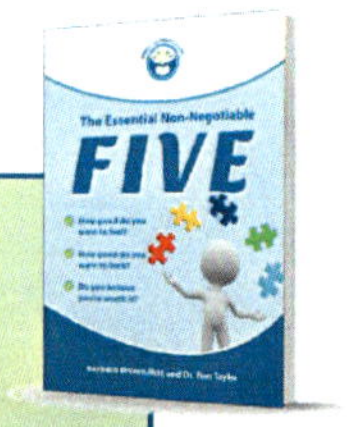

The Essential, Non-Negotiable Five

1. **TRACE MINERALS PLUS+®** plant-based liquid minerals
2. **JUICE PLUS+®** 30 Fruits, Veggies, & grains in capsules!
3. **ASEA®** immune-boosting "redox signaling" supplement
4. **ALKALINE IONIZED WATER**, antioxidizing and truly hydrating!
5. **BARBARA'S ULTIMATE POWER SHAKE** Satisfying & delicious!

You'll find these and every other nutritional product featured in ***Your Personal Roadmap to Whole Body Cleansing***, along with specific remedies, everything you'll need for all the cleanses, and other tools too, at our web site below:

www.CLEANSINGROADMAP.com

NOTE: ***All of the products we refer to throughout the book are the same ones we use ourselves.*** We have tested them extensively, found them to be the best available, and have recommended them to clients for years, with consistently positive results. Our guiding principle for taking or recommending any product is...

> ***"It doesn't matter what you take.***
> ***It matters what your body does with what you take."***
> **Dr. Tom Taylor**

The only products we use or recommend are those that withstand our "100% test":

1. The body must be able to *recognize, absorb* and *utilize* the product.
2. It must provide *superior benefit* with little or *no added stress* to the body.
3. It must always test strong on kinesiological or energetic testing *(aka, "muscle testing," see page 106)* for anyone, at any age and in any condition. Any product that tests weak is excluded immediately.

Take advantage of the online resources for this book at

YourPremiumWBC.wl-wh.com

If you ordered from Amazon:

Please first register your purchase at registerWBC.wl-wh.com

Many of the products in these pages may be purchased at "member" prices directly from the companies that market them. We may receive compensation from these companies as a result of your purchase. Earnings go to support non-profit ministries that help restore broken lives.

"Your body is a stimulus-response mechanism.

If you want a different response, change the stimulus that makes the response necessary."

"No amount of treatment will correct a nutritional deficiency."

Dr. Tom Taylor

Why Bother?

Imagine how you would look and feel on the outside if you'd never taken a shower: layer upon layer of dust, dirt, grease and grime, packed over your skin, unable to breathe or take in water...*YUCK!* Believe it or not, your insides may look a lot like that! Scary thought, isn't it?

It's not only possible but proven that stubborn weight can be *eliminated*; so can allergies, acid reflux and persistent fatigue! Failing memories can *improve* and thinning bones can be *rebuilt*! Amazingly, even the spirit within you can be renewed, enabling you to fulfill your life's purpose with energy and delight!

When you decide to clean the gunk out of your insides, you begin a liberating adventure to unload the "gunk" you've accumulated, and discover how good your body, mind, and spirit can feel!

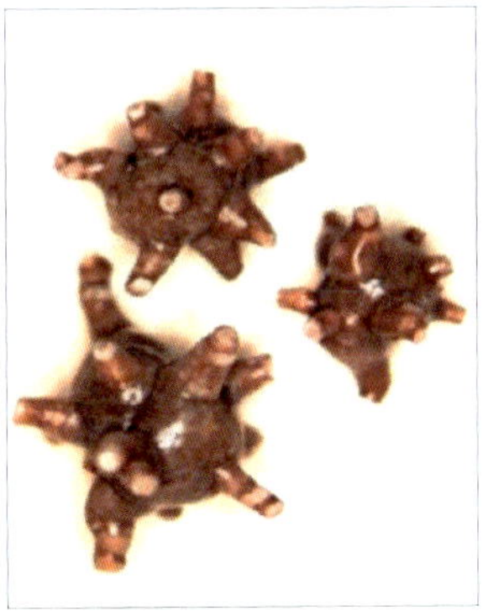

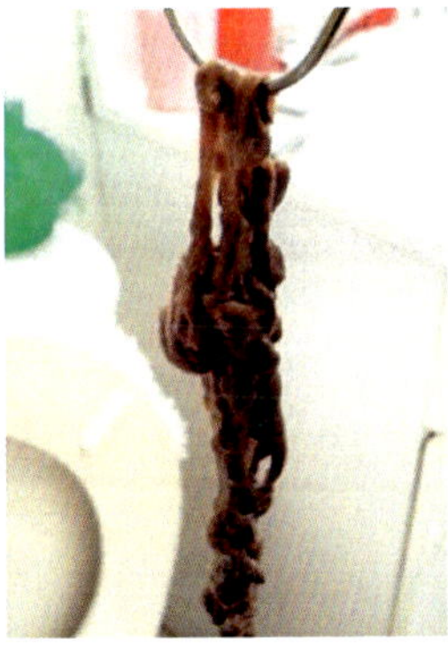

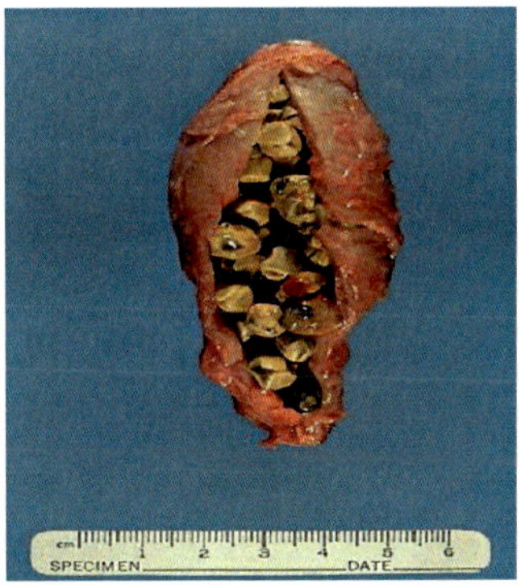

These are actual photos (from left to right) of kidney stones, colon "sludge," and a gallbladder full of stones. Not pretty, is it? Yet the people who had these "treasures" may have thought they were perfectly healthy!

Within a few short weeks of beginning your first cleanse, the difference in how you feel will astonish you in ways it's impossible to appreciate until you begin!

A Short Trip from the Mouth South

Believe it or not, the 12 meter-long (39.4 feet) "tube" from the mouth to the rectum – the "alimentary canal" – is considered to be *outside* your body. The digestive tract, including the esophagus, stomach, small intestine (or small bowel), and large intestine (aka, the colon), is one long, open tube. Everything you eat and drink runs *through* your body, literally, north to south.

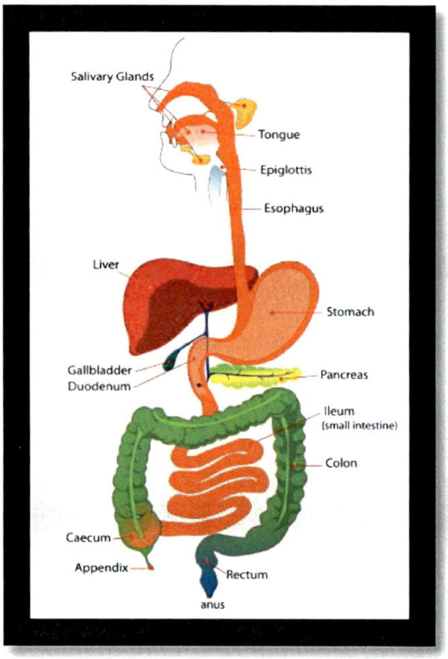

The digestive system is responsible for breaking down food into usable nutrients and eliminating the waste. Think of it as one big processing plant. You put stuff in and different stuff comes out!

The higher the quality of what you eat and drink, the better everything inside you works, the healthier you are, and the better you feel. Your diet affects *everything*: energy, mood, memory, movement, life span...you name it!

Bottom line: How healthy you are depends, in large part, on what you eat and drink...what you put in. How well you feel and how good you look depends on how well everything inside you deals with what you eat and drink.

How well do you want to feel?

How good do you want to look?

Do you believe you're worth it?

THE SIMPLE TRUTH ABOUT HEALTHY CLEANSING

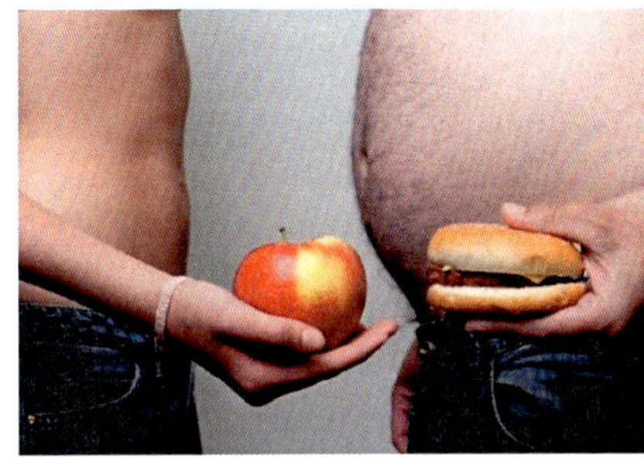

You probably brush your teeth twice a day, but when was the last time you "brushed" your liver, gallbladder, or colon? When was the last time you hosed down your kidneys or wrung out your pancreas? Think about it: We're putting food and liquids through these organs every day. It might be time to "get the gunk out" and run your digestive system through a "wash cycle," unless you've eaten raw food all your life.

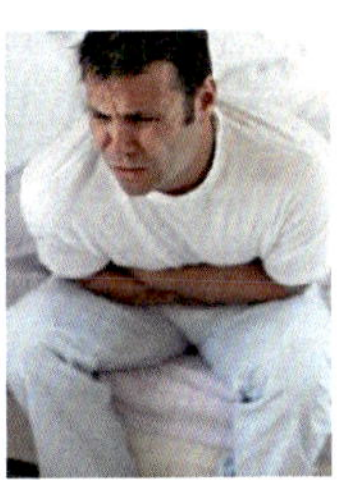

Many chronic health problems originate with faulty digestion, absorption and elimination caused by a digestive tract that has become caked with residue accumulated through years of poor elimination and a diet of processed foods. Residue around the walls of the colon can become hardened or rubbery, forming a "pipe," which interferes with the transfer of waste materials and the absorption of nutrients. When these vital processes are impeded we become malnourished and toxic, leading to disease and weight issues. A healthy digestive tract is the foundation of a healthy body.

Cleansing is perfectly safe when it is approached carefully and performed methodically, allowing the body to heal throughout the process.

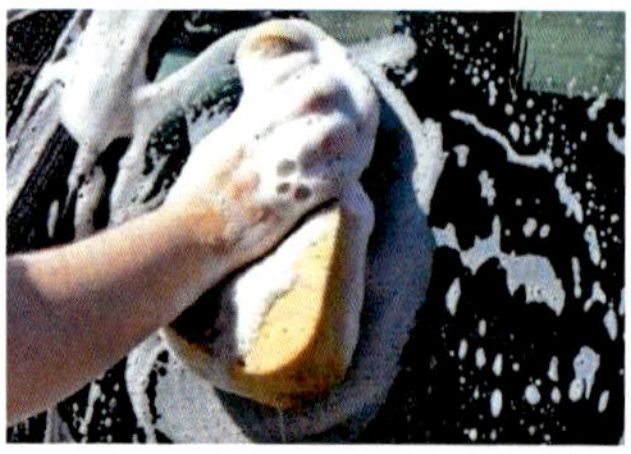

Not all cleanses are created equal. The most effective ones we have found help *"decongest," rejuvenate, and revitalize* organs over time and in a logical order: liver, kidneys, gallbladder, and colon. Along the way, the stomach, pancreas, heart, adrenals, thyroid, and brain – virtually every cell in the body – benefits. The entire process is designed to improve enzyme production and movement of materials through the digestive process; restore nutrient-absorbing and waste-eliminating functions, return the intestinal tract to its proper environment; and correct the overall body chemistry (pH balance).

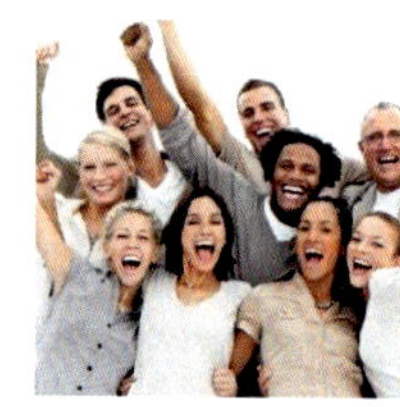

EFFECTIVE CLEANSING PROGRAMS USE MANY COMMON ELEMENTS:

- **A material to "scrape"** hardened material off the colon walls. We use CLEAN SWEEP MIX™ (see page 36 for the recipe), a proprietary, all-organic mix of soluble and insoluble fiber to encourage bowel motility, move debris through the digestive tract and out for good; plus, power greens to nourish your cells at the same time!
- **A bowel regulator** such as whole-leaf aloe vera juice, raw fruit juices, organic blackstrap molasses, or an herb, like *cascara sagrada*.
- **Liquid minerals** to support efficient chemical reactions in every cell, promote healing of the tissues, and kill microscopic parasites.
- **Probiotics** to re-establish healthy bacteria in the intestines.
- **DETOX CLAY** — Liquid Bentonite to bind and eliminate excess toxins.
- **Water** — lots of it — to flush the system.
- **Whole food concentrates**, such as fruit, vegetable and berry powder in capsules, barley grass, or other green powders, can help cleanse, rebuild, and support every cell in your body for the rest of your life.
- **Digestive enzymes** to help the stomach and pancreas work more easily and efficiently; reduce gas, bloating, burping, and indigestion.

> **Making sudden or drastic changes in your eating habits is not always advisable; check with a competent holistic health care practitioner, or contact us directly for help.**

When deciding to go through whole body cleansing for the first time, you may want to begin slowly, adding vegetables, fruit and whole grains to your diet over a period of as much as six weeks, to replace processed foods you may be used to eating. As you gradually introduce more whole foods, your body will adapt to a higher quality diet.

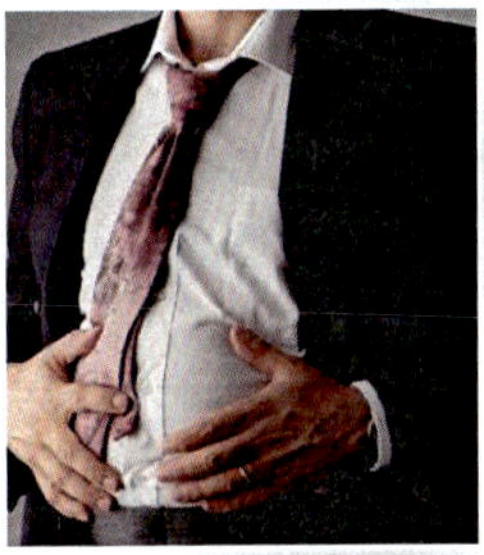

You may experience some abdominal bloating or gas. This is a sign that the pancreas is failing to produce sufficient enzymes. We recommend an enzyme supplement, called DAILY ENZYME COMPLEX, to help supply the necessary enzymes, while taking the load off the pancreas to enable this vital gland to renew itself. The number of tablets needed may vary from two to six or even more, taken within an hour or two after meals. You'll find more on this subject on page 14.

If burping or "heartburn" symptoms occur, VEGETARIAN ENZYME COMPLEX is the recommended supplement to help the stomach digest its contents more efficiently. Take two to six tablets with meals.

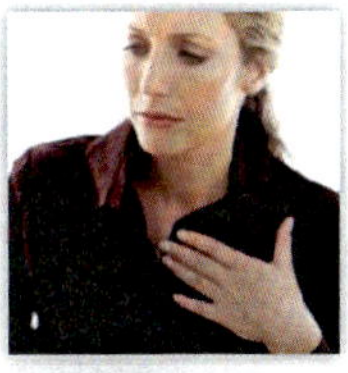

If constipation occurs, the **SALTWATER FLUSH** on page 53 is an excellent way to help gently but effectively stimulate the bowels. If needed, you may use the herb, *Cascara Sagrada*, until the bowels move easily two to three times per day. CLEAN SWEEP MIX™ in the cleanses we discuss later should be cut in half until the problem resolves.

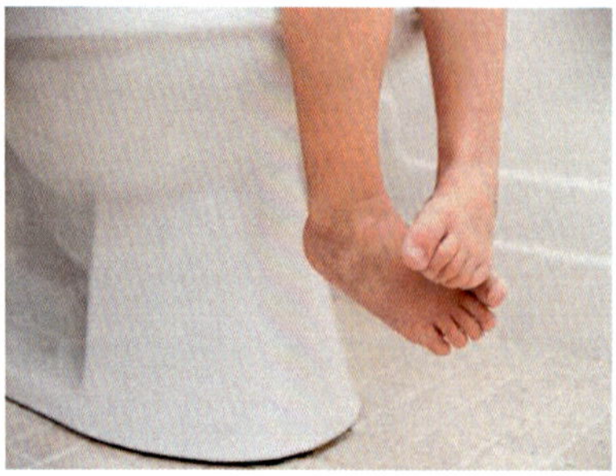

There will likely be changes in your elimination. *This means that you will actually have to look!* Most people are amazed at what they unknowingly carried in their colons. Changes in color, texture and frequency of your stool are desired results. You should be able to *see* that you are eliminating layers of old "stuff." The proof is in the toilet!

During a cleanse, you may experience short periods of symptoms such as headaches, body aches, nausea, or flu-like symptoms. This simply indicates that you are stirring up and eliminating old toxins.

Most intestinal cleanses need to be performed consistently for at least three months to achieve the best results.

We have used most of the cleanses presented here ourselves and have supervised countless others through their processes successfully. The feeling of rejuvenation is well worth the effort. Surgeries have been avoided and even lives have been saved!

Chronic diarrhea or constipation should be brought to your health practitioner's attention.

It's time to get your insides squeaky clean and learn how to live well in the body God gave you!

Let's get to it …

The more determined you are, the better your results will be.

Your health is your choice!

First Things First
Rejuvenate Your Liver

The first organ to clean is *not the colon*, it's the liver! Next to the skin, the liver is the largest organ in the body. It is the major site of detoxification (the process of removing "poisons" such as alcohol, drugs and food additives).

Cleaning out the colon *before* the liver can efficiently process the toxins being released into the blood stream may create more problems than it solves!

Among many other functions, the liver produces bile to break down dietary fats; converts glucose to glycogen (a form of stored sugar); makes amino acids (protein building blocks); stores vitamins A, D, K and B12; and maintains proper blood glucose levels. Most people think the pancreas regulates blood sugar, but the liver does as much as 70 percent of the job, and also produces around 90 percent of the cholesterol your body uses.

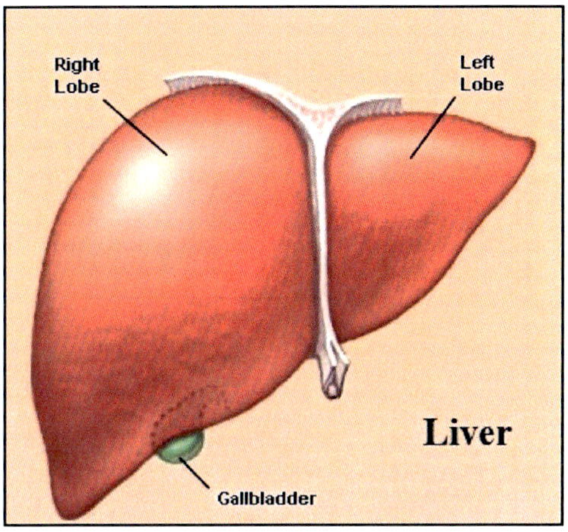

Rejuvenating the liver helps your whole body to work more efficiently. Every organ and gland – heart, brain, adrenals, thyroid, kidneys, etc. – depends on a healthy liver.

Rejuvenating the liver is an excellent "kick-start" to change from being a fat-storing to a fat-burning machine! Foods that facilitate this process are low in protein (especially from animal sources). This relieves everyday stress on the liver and avoids the unhealthy burden on the liver that high-protein diets create.

Busting the Cholesterol Myth

Despite reports to the contrary, cholesterol is neither good nor bad...it is *essential* for building hormones, Vitamin D, cell membranes, and bile acids that digest fat. Cholesterol makes up about 60 percent of the brain and is critical for proper neurological function.

According to leading experts, there is no such thing as "good cholesterol" or "bad cholesterol." Even the long-held notion that high cholesterol levels contribute to heart disease has been repudiated.

Ron Rosedale, MD, is considered a leading expert in the field of anti-aging. Here's some of what he says about cholesterol:

> **"Cholesterol is a vital component of every cell membrane on Earth. That fact alone tells you that in and of itself, it cannot be evil; in fact, it is one of your best friends. You would not be here without it. No wonder that lowering cholesterol too much artificially increases your risk of dying."**

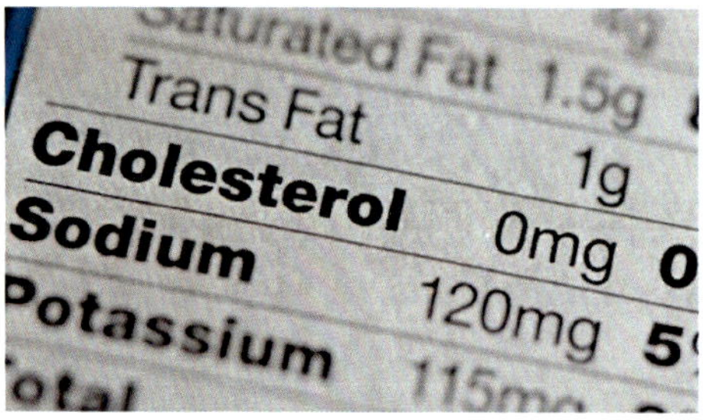

Dr. Rosedale and other experts note that cholesterol does not create plaque in the arteries; rather, oxidized fats, called "lipid peroxides" are the culprits. In a 1996 study, published in the Journal of Current Therapeutic Research, a whole-food based nutritional product, JUICE PLUS+®, lowered "lipid peroxides" (rancid fats) by 75 percent or more in only 28 days. At the same time, important antioxidants, such as tocopherols, selenium, zeaxanthin, and others, along with critical minerals such as calcium, were significantly increased; all without changing any other dietary or other habits.

Rejuvenate Your Liver in 14 Days

Within only three days of beginning the liver rejuvenating program, your over-stimulated sugar receptors are "re-set" and your body will begin burning fat as fuel, rather than sugar. Cravings may come and go during this time; however, people often report fewer cravings, especially for sweets, by the time they complete the program.

You'll begin to realize the difference between "hunger" (what you *need)* and "appetite" (what you *reach for*).

If you're a caffeine-drinker, you may notice some tiredness, but this should last only one or two days. By the fourth day of the program, as the liver decongests and fat is made more available for energy, you should begin to feel more energetic and sleep will become deeper.

DON'T SKIP MEALS! You'll be eating more than enough at meal time and in between to feel satisfied, but it's important to eat throughout the program.

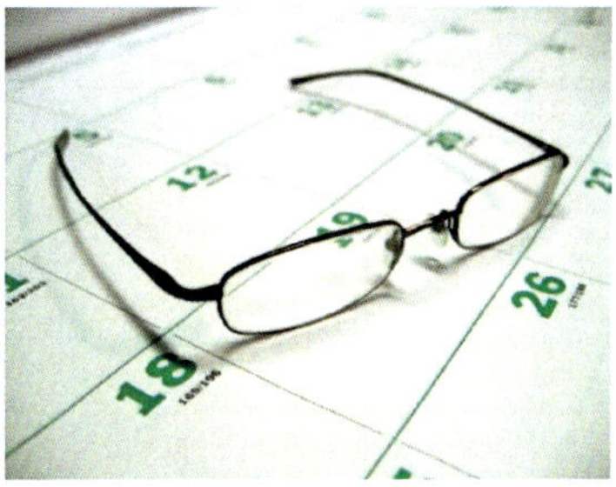

You may begin to eliminate excess weight and inches during the 14 days. Other benefits include improvements in skin and nails, flexibility, fewer aches and pains, and even increased sex drive.

You're welcome to continue the liver rejuvenating program beyond the first two weeks. It is both safe and even advisable to eat this way for as long as you feel well, aren't craving protein, and aren't fatiguing easily. After the first two weeks, you may add a *small* amount of animal protein each day.

Some people may need to add a little animal protein during the first two weeks. Fatigue, light-headedness, lethargy, feeling cold, and cravings for protein are signs that more protein may be needed.

The symptoms above are due mainly to poor blood sugar regulation. As little as 10 grams of protein (fish or eggs) added per day – *not per meal* – is usually enough to resolve the symptoms.

If necessary, small amounts of protein may be added daily until the symptoms disappear; protein can then be decreased slowly or even eliminated.

Other cleanses may be combined with the liver rejuvenating program to begin working on other body systems. A list of these cleanses and our recommended sequence to follow to achieve the best results can be found on pages 99-100.

Bloated?

Burping or abdominal bloating and gas may result from adding raw vegetables to the diet too quickly (or even cooked vegetables, if you aren't used to them). The stomach and pancreas may not make sufficient enzymes to break down complex carbohydrates efficiently. Diets high in processed foods tend to deplete or suppress the body's enzyme-making system, but that capacity will be rebuilt over time as you follow a series of cleansing processes.

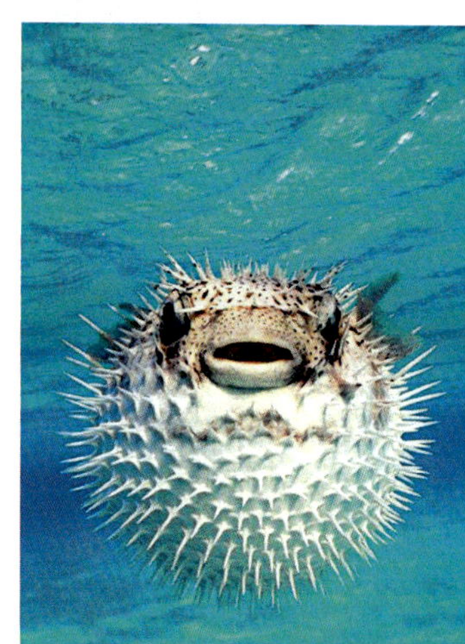

If bloating occurs, take 1-3 DAILY ENZYME COMPLEX tablets about an hour after meals. You can avoid some vegetables temporarily, such as asparagus, beans, broccoli, Brussels sprouts, cauliflower, carrots, cabbage, cucumbers, green beans, green peppers, lettuce, onions, and radishes, until your body is better able to tolerate them. Avoiding these foods is limiting, and certainly not ideal, but is still workable.

How Rejuvenating the Liver Works

Rejuvenating the liver is more of a healing process than a true cleanse, sort of like getting rid of a cold. Over the next 14 days, your liver will be "decongesting," recuperating, and re-establishing efficient operations. This is an important starting point for other cleanses that follow, which will also benefit the liver.

While on this program, you will consume lots of greens, little fat, and minimal animal protein (unless your blood sugar gets too low, as discussed earlier). Refined or processed foods, and starchy foods like potatoes, breads and pasta, should be avoided. Lists of foods to emphasize or avoid are included in the following pages.

"What can I eat?" is the most common question we're asked. The answer to that and other questions may be found on the next several pages. We've also provided some menu ideas.

Eat mostly raw and lightly cooked, nutrient-dense vegetables. The more colorful the better!

Cruciferous vegetables (the ones starred in the chart on page 17) are among the healthiest foods for the liver. They contain cancer-fighting properties and, together with other nutrient-dense vegetables, will help decongest and rejuvenate your liver the fastest.

Since fat readily satisfies hunger, and this program is relatively low in fat, eat more food more frequently!

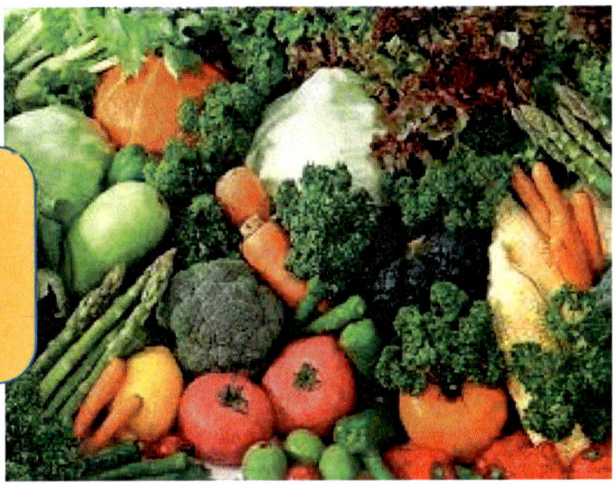

DRINK THIS BEFORE EVERY MEAL:
Cranberry-Vinegar-Lemon Drink

Mix the following liquids together, according to the following recipe, to facilitate and accelerate the process of rejuvenating the liver:

- **8 oz.** Alkaline Ionized, reverse osmosis, or filtered water.
- **2 oz. Unsweetened Cranberry Juice** supports the body's filtration system: liver, kidneys, bladder and urinary tract. Pure juices can be found at health food stores and in the natural food section of most supermarkets.

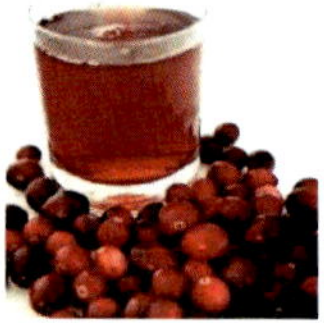

- **½-1 teaspoon Apple Cider Vinegar** (non-distilled) helps reduce water retention by normalizing the body's acid and alkaline balance (pH), eliminates waste acids, and provides alkalizing minerals like organic potassium and sodium. It also fortifies the friendly bacteria in the intestines. Adjust the amount to taste.

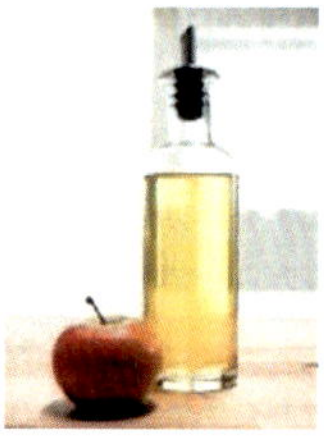

- **1 Tablespoon Lemon Juice** (fresh squeezed) has astringent properties to aid in decongesting the liver, and supports immune function. Use up to a whole lemon if you have a history of kidney stones.

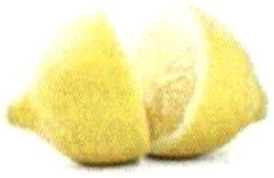

- **Mix enough for a full day and refrigerate.**

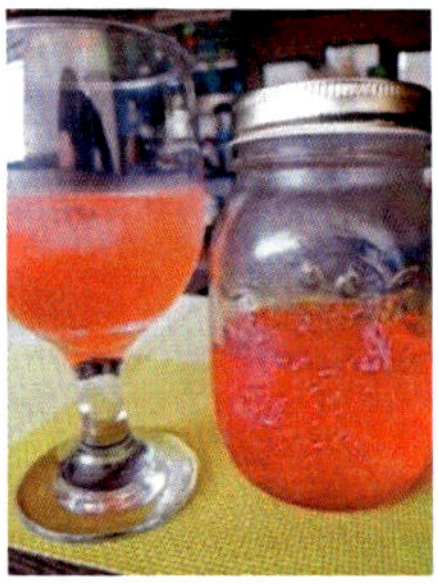

OPTIONAL:

- **Apple juice** (no more than ¼ cup). Use this *only* if you can't stand the taste of the Cranberry-Vinegar-Lemon drink.
- **Fiber** (1-2 Tbsp) to help curb hunger. CLEAN SWEEP MIX™ (page 36) is recommended for this and other cleanses. Add it just before drinking as the fiber swells quickly.

This may not be the most delicious drink you've ever tasted, but most people tolerate it well for 14 days. If you just can't stand the taste, reduce the amount of vinegar or eliminate it altogether.

You Can't Overdose on Vegetables, So Eat 'em Up!

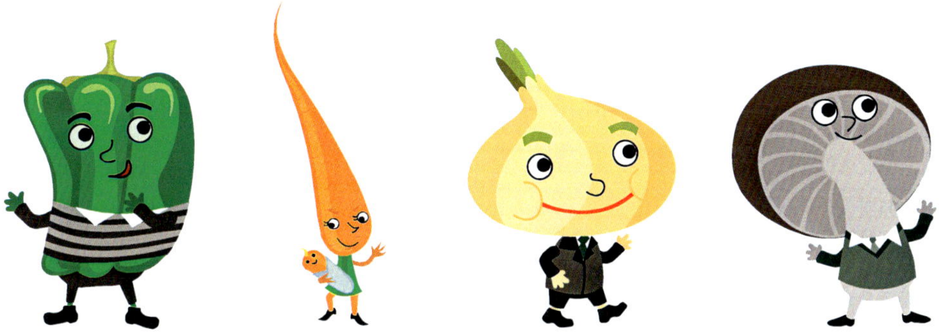

Eat as many different kinds as possible!

The list below is by no means complete, but illustrates the variety available:

• artichokes	• cauliflower*	• lettuce (not iceberg!)	• seaweed (Nori)
• asparagus	• celery	• mushrooms	• spinach
• avocado	• collard greens*	• okra	• squash
• green beans	• corn**	• olives	• string beans
• beets	• cucumbers	• onions	• snap peas
• bok choy* (Chinese cabbage)	• eggplant	• parsley	• sprouts – all
• broccoli*	• garlic	• peas, peapods	• Swiss chard
• Brussels sprouts*	• jicama	• peppers (all)	• tomatoes***
• cabbage*	• kale*	• radishes*	• turnips and turnip greens*
• carrots	• leeks	• sauerkraut	• zucchini

* Cruciferous vegetables

** Corn may also be classified as a grain. Eat it young, fresh or frozen.

*** Tomatoes are also considered fruit.

Cruciferous vegetables in the chart on the previous page have a slight tendency to reduce iodine, a trace element used for producing thyroid hormones. Nevertheless, eating as many cruciferous vegetables as possible is recommended because of their ability to help improve the function of the liver.

If you take thyroid medication, add foods that contain iodine, like seaweed, navy beans, straw-berries, molasses, and sea salt.

In addition to the foods above, some of the nutritional supplements on pages 27-28 will prevent iodine deficiency.

For maximum nutrition, the best way to eat vegetables is raw. Cooked vegetables are best lightly sautéed or steamed. The smell of cooked food comes from the contents of the actual plant cells breaking open over heat. Remove vegetables from the stove when you smell them cooking to avoid destroying delicate enzymes and vitamins.

At least half of the vegetables in your diet should be eaten raw. Even frozen, organically grown vegetables are excellent, because they are picked ripe, cleaned and frozen quickly, preserving most of the enzyme and vitamin content.

Eat as many vegetables and as large a variety as you can, including snacks between meals. The benefits of the high nutrient density in vegetables cannot be over-emphasized.

You can't eat too many vegetables, so *Go For It!*

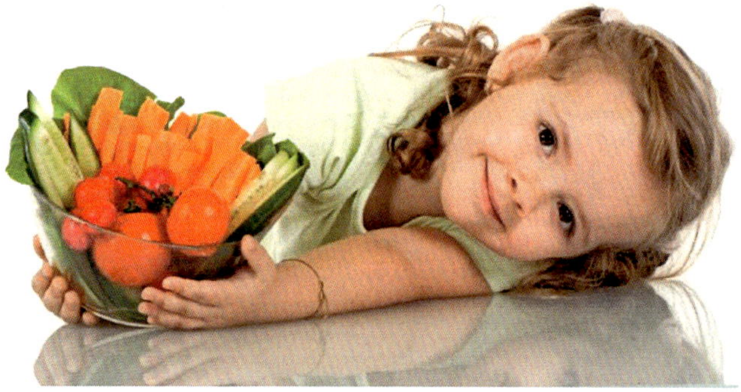

Two Vegetable Superfood Superstars

Walk down any well-stocked produce aisle and pick two – just two – of the most nutrient-dense, vitamin-loaded vegetables to take home to your family. What would they be? Carrots? Good choice. Peppers? Excellent. Broccoli? Sure. Spinach? You're getting warm.

KALE IS KING. Not many people really like kale, but it is a superior vegetable because of its amazing nutrient density. Kale may be lightly steamed or served raw in salad, by itself or with other greens. It is *slightly* bitter, so adding shredded carrots, parsnips, beets, sprouts, and almonds helps improve the flavor.

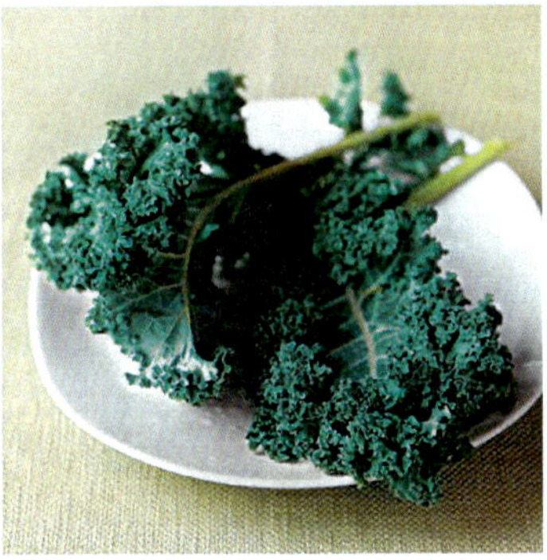

Kale is one of the best sources of organic minerals such as calcium, potassium and manganese, as well as vitamins A and C. In addition, kale contains cancer-fighting nutrients such as indole-3-carbinol, a compound that activates enzymes in the liver which help neutralize potential carcinogens in the diet.

SPROUTS ARE SPECTACULAR. Nutrients in small quantities of sprouts are equivalent to those found in large amounts of mature vegetables. Sprouts are readily available in supermarkets and are also easy to grow at home with commercially available sprouting jars. For maximum benefit, add sprouts daily to salads. They are essential in your diet!

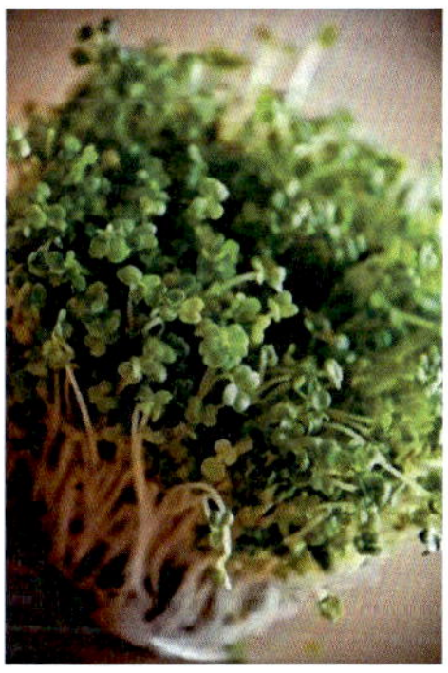

One ounce of broccoli sprouts contains 20-50 times more enzyme-induced activity (anti-cancer properties) than mature, cooked broccoli.

A Few Guidelines

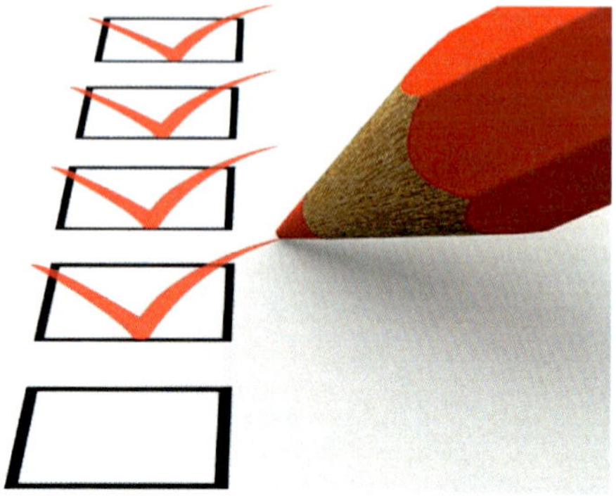

1. **Stick to the lists of recommended foods.** Sugar and hidden sugars in juices, sport drinks, protein bars, flavored yogurt, etc. can slow down the healing process dramatically.
2. **Drink plenty of water:** 64 to 80 ounces per day. Alkaline Ionized Water is superior, but water filtered by reverse osmosis is acceptable. Avoid drinking tap water. Herbal tea is permitted.
3. **Avoid caffeine.** If you feel easily fatigued, or suffer withdrawal symptoms such as headaches, drink only enough to resolve the symptoms. Blend decaffeinated with regular coffee until none is needed. If possible, use organic, water-process decaffeinated coffee.
4. **The liver rejuvenating process can be repeated or extended** to keep the liver in top shape. Some people continue the program for several months.
5. **Exercise with caution** if your energy is low. Make sure to keep your pulse rate below 130.
6. **Avoid dairy.** As noted previously, a *small* amount of low-fat cottage cheese, plain low-fat yogurt, a little butter, and low-fat cheese is acceptable, though not ideal.
7. **Avoid anything with MSG** (monosodium glutamate). This flavor-enhancer is a stimulant and a toxin to the nervous system. It also stimulates the appetite, which is why it's difficult to stop eating many snack foods, and why we feel hungry soon after eating Chinese food.

Steer Clear of Starches and Grains

Starch is really just sugar in a more complex form; likewise for grains; plus, the gluten contained in grains presents other unnecessary challenges. Starches and other sugars seriously hamper the process of rejuvenating the liver. Here are some specific starches to avoid:

- **Potatoes** (white or sweet, including fries & chips)
- **Breads** (including bagels)
- **Donuts and Pastries** (includes croissants, muffins, and pancakes)
- **Pasta and Rice**
- **Cereal, Crackers, Rice Cakes**
- **Anything made from the foods listed above**
- **Alcohol,** even as little as a few ounces of wine will stop the rejuvenation for three days!

MILLET is one grain that may be used *sparingly*. Quinoa is a seed related to spinach. Both are alkaline-producing, like vegetables and almonds (other grains are acid-forming). You'll find millet and quinoa at most better supermarkets.

Sacrifice the Sacred Cow

We could devote an entire book to this subject, but for now let's just say that dairy products are extremely mucus-producing, contain a protein that humans can't digest, aren't the best source of calcium by a long shot, are congestive to the liver, and should be avoided.

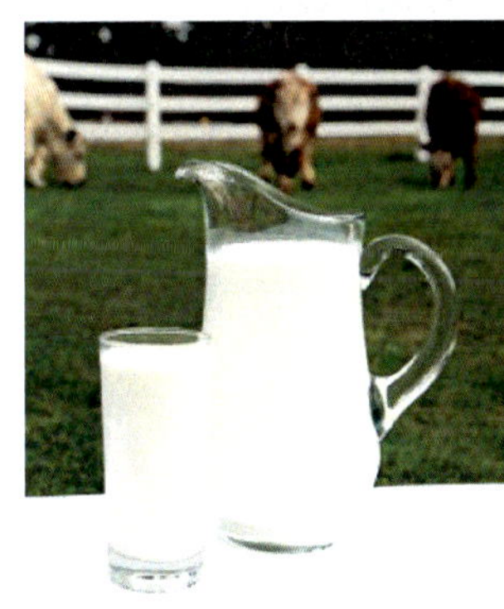

EXCEPTIONS: A little feta cheese sprinkled on salad; cottage cheese, plain low-fat yogurt, and butter in *small* amounts (no more than 6 oz. total per day). Occasionally, yogurt cheese (3 oz. at most) may be tolerated.

Salad Dressings

Use just enough of any dressing to flavor the salad. Making your own dressing is the healthiest choice. Try mixing balsamic or apple cider vinegar, olive oil and your own spices.

If you opt for bottled dressing, we offer three words of advice:

Read the Labels!

Many bottled salad dressings contain sugars, high-fructose corn syrup, food colors, or other chemicals that make the liver work harder than necessary. Health food stores or local supermarkets with natural food sections should have a variety of healthy dressings from which to choose.

MSG, (monosodium glutamate), also known as modified food starch, must be avoided! It is very detrimental to the liver.

TURMERIC: A spice with an astonishing list of health benefits, well worth reading about (see George Mateljan Foundation and WHFoods.org). Sprinkle this orange-colored spice on both raw and cooked vegetables daily.

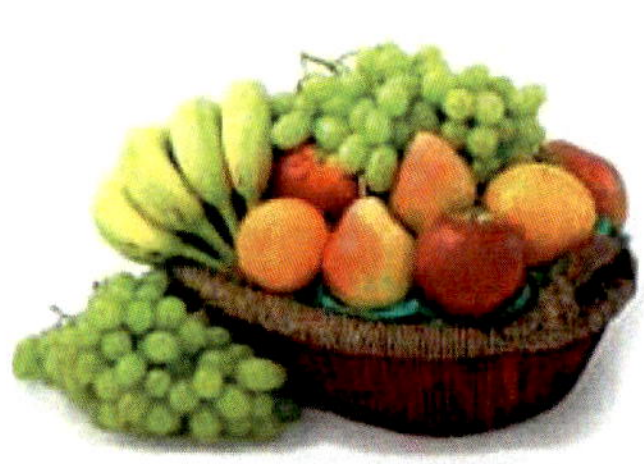

Fruit

Half a cup of berries or other fruit is a great snack, but eat only one third as many fruits as total vegetables (1 cup of vegetables to 1/3 cup of fruit). Mixing in low-fat cottage cheese or plain yogurt helps slow the release of sugar into the blood stream. High-fiber fruit also slows sugar absorption and the release of insulin, a powerful fat-storing hormone. Fruit juices, bananas, dates, figs, raisins, other dried or canned fruit should be avoided. You may find that eating fruit in the morning leads to cravings for sweets or other foods, fatigue or low endurance.

Grapefruit has been shown to increase the potency of some medications. Check with your doctor, or avoid grapefruit if you are taking medication.

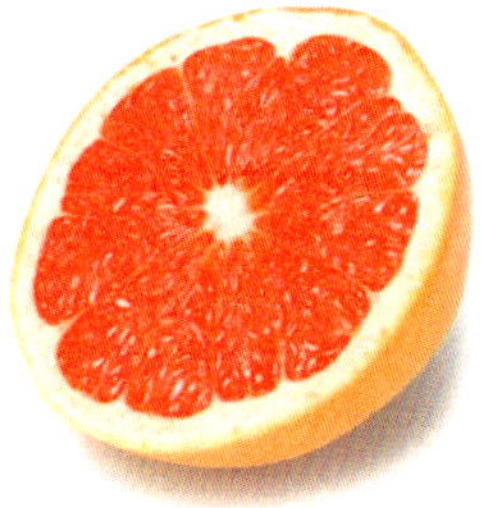

Here's a list of some recommended fruits:

- **Apples, berries and kiwi**
- **Apricots, plums and grapes**
- **Grapefruit, oranges, lemons and limes**
- **Nectarines, peaches and pears**
- **Cherries and pineapple (small amounts)**

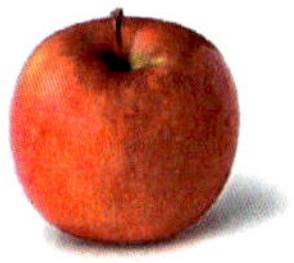

Apples Are the Exception to the "No Fruit Rule"

- Apples are high in alkalizing minerals such as potassium and calcium.
- They are high in fiber, which slows the body's insulin response and helps regulate blood sugar.
- Malic acid in apples is an excellent solvent for stagnant bile in the liver.
- Apples contain gelatin-like pectin, which can help lower cholesterol.
- Apples may lower the incidence of cancer.
(French National Institute for Health and Medical Research)

Apples may be eaten anytime and in any amount!

Animal Protein

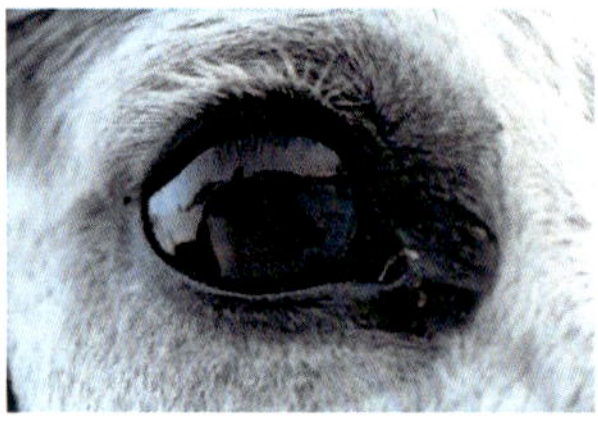

Anything that has eyes, whether it runs, crawls, flies, swims, or slithers, is considered animal protein. It takes a great deal of energy in the liver to process animal protein and it should be avoided for at least the first two weeks.

There is no risk of becoming protein deficient! However, if you experience low blood sugar symptoms (light-headedness, dizziness, difficulty concentrating, excessive fatigue, feeling cold, hair loss, or uncontrollable cravings for protein), add a *small* amount of one of the choices below:

- **Fish** – Wild caught *(not farm-raised)* cod, haddock, halibut, salmon, tuna, sea bass, or trout. These should be baked or broiled. Raw, sushi-grade is also good, but it must be fresh!
- **Eggs** – Farm fresh is always best. Organic, free-range and cage-free are also good choices.
- **Chicken, turkey, ostrich, lamb, buffalo or beef** – grass-fed, free-range or organic meats are best. "Natural" meats are free of growth hormones and/or antibiotics, but are still usually fed a diet that is not natural to the animal.

Start with one egg per day (hard-boiled, soft-boiled or poached) or a small piece of fish (2-3 ounces). Eggs and fish put the least amount of stress on the liver, because they are less acid-forming and easier to digest than other meats.

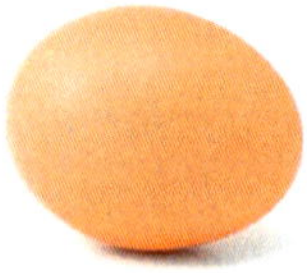

CAUTION: Overeating protein is easy to do and it stresses the liver. To avoid this, eat small amounts frequently, and just enough to satisfy your hunger. Any symptoms related to having less protein in your diet will disappear as the liver regains its health.

Nuts and Seeds

THE GOOD NEWS: Pound for pound, nuts and seeds are incredibly dense packets of high quality protein, vitamins, minerals and essential fats. Eating raw nuts, seeds and hummus (made with chickpeas) is important to prevent hunger between meals. **Raw almonds** and **Brazil nuts** are best because both are alkalizing (the importance of alkalizing foods is discussed on pages 57-58, and 65).

Dipping sliced apples in almond butter is a great treat. Although natural, organic peanut butter is allowed, **almond butter is a far superior choice.**

In addition to almonds and Brazil nuts, here are some good choices:

- Cashews
- Pistachios
- Pecans
- Walnuts
- Pine nuts
- Sunflower seeds
- Sesame seeds

THE BAD NEWS: Nuts, seeds and most grains contain *enzyme inhibitors*, which naturally prevent growth until the right condition exists for germination in the soil.

Enzyme inhibitors, such as phytic acid, may block the absorption of iron, calcium, copper, magnesium, and zinc in the intestinal tract. The pancreas may also exhaust its enzymes trying to overcome these inhibitors. The result may be gas, bloating, slower digestion generally, and more difficulty in processing *all* foods. People often mistake this condition for a food sensitivity or allergy.

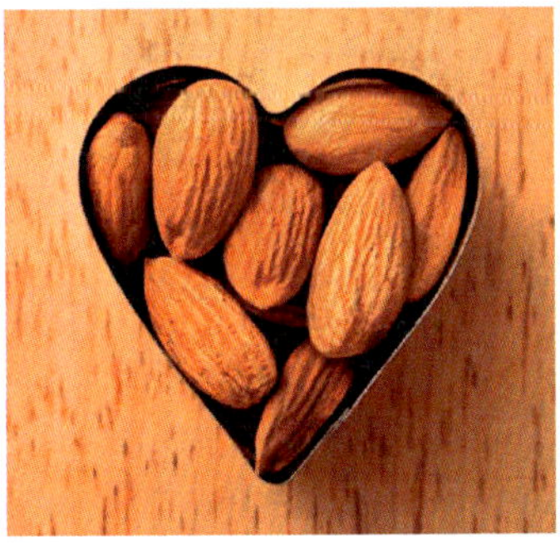

Studies have found a doubling in the size of the pancreas, along with stunted growth, impaired health, and decreased enzyme reserves, when animals are fed nuts or seeds without de-activating the enzyme inhibitors.

Peanuts Aren't Really Nuts!

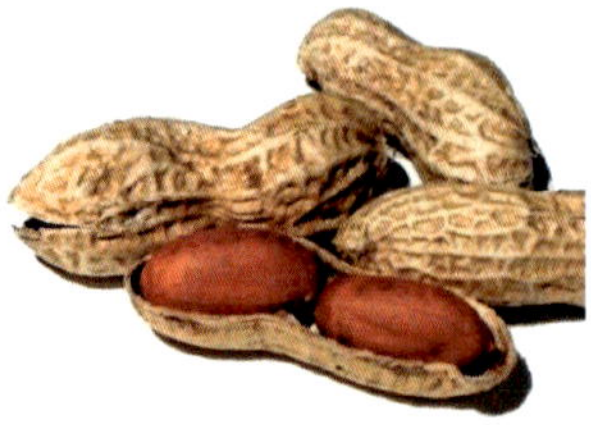

Peanuts are actually legumes, like beans and peas, all of which produce seed pods and grow on vines, not trees. Peanuts also contain *aflatoxins*, which may be carcinogenic in humans. Many people have allergic reactions to peanuts, which may even be life-threatening.

Solution: Germinate Nuts and Seeds

Germinate means "to cause to sprout or grow"

Germinating nuts and seeds preserves their dense nutritional value, and unlocks natural enzyme activity to help nuts and seeds become more easily digested. Germinating can reduce, or even prevent, bloating and allergic reactions.

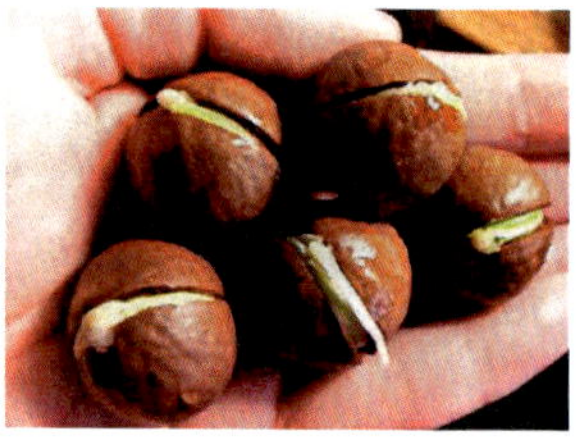

HERE'S HOW TO DO IT:

1. Soak seeds and nuts in filtered water overnight *(12 hours)*. Use a glass or metal container covered with cheesecloth or other breathable fabric.
2. In the morning, rinse and drain the freshly germinated seeds and nuts several times, to wash off the enzyme inhibitors.
3. Let germinated nuts and seeds dry thoroughly, and keep them in the refrigerator until eaten, because they will spoil quicker. If you have more than a 4 to 5-day supply, use a dehydrator to remove any remaining water content. *(Set dehydrator no higher than 105 degrees F for 18–24 hours. Remember, enzymes are very sensitive to heat)*.
4. ENJOY! This is live "*superfood*" with lots of nutrition that your body can actually use!
5. Refrigerate any leftover nuts or seeds in a glass container.

Germinate Beans and Lentils, Except One

Beans and lentils, like nuts, should be soaked overnight to release their enzyme inhibitors before cooking, for easier digestion and maximum nutrition. Sprouting also makes nutrients in beans and lentils more readily available.

Processed beans, such as refried and baked beans, are not recommended.

NEVER SPROUT KIDNEY BEANS!

They must be germinated and then fully cooked to destroy a naturally occurring toxin, and to make them digestible.

Nutritional Supplements

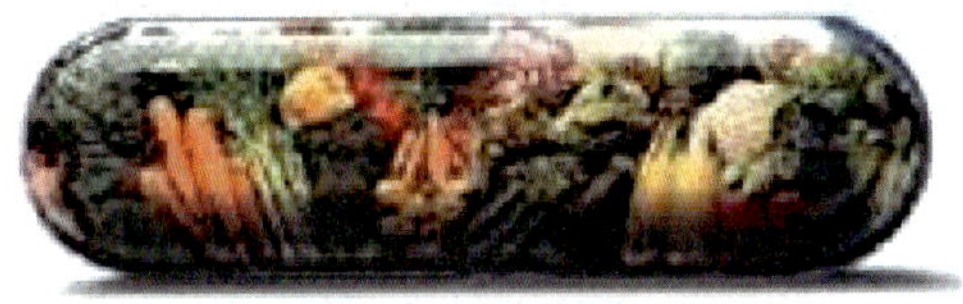

The truth is that food — even when it is organically grown — cannot supply all of the nutrients we need to thrive. Nutritional supplementation is an essential part of any wellness lifestyle. Studies show that whole-food concentrates deliver a complete spectrum of vitamins, antioxidants, and other *phytonutrients* (nutrients that are naturally contained in plants). Unlike vitamin formulas, nutrients in whole-food concentrates are naturally synergistic; our bodies *recognize* them, *absorb* them easily, and, most importantly, *utilize* them efficiently. Whole-food supplements provide a nutritional safety net to bridge the gap between what we *should* do and what we *really* do every day!

For information about specific whole-food nutritional products we use and recommend, go to www.CleansingRoadmap.com

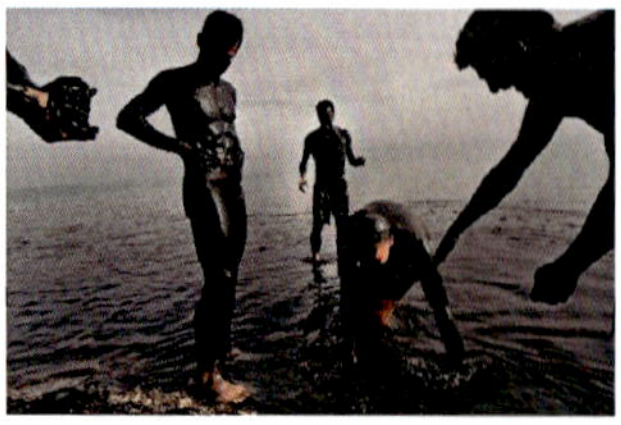

Don't Forget Your Minerals

Minerals have been known for their healing properties for thousands of years. Native Americans would heal wounds by packing them with clay from a riverbed. Over a million people enjoy "mud baths" in the Dead Sea every year, and millions more flock to natural mineral baths around the world. Silver coins were often dropped into pioneer canteens and water barrels to prevent bacterial growth. Minerals such as calcium, magnesium, potassium, iodine, and iron are well known, but what you may not know is that there are more than 72 major minerals and trace elements, most of which are unavailable in foods today, because our soils have been depleted of these important minerals since the advent of modern farming methods in the early 1900s. Mineral deficiencies are rampant and can have more serious health consequences than you realize.

Minerals are essential to life itself. Every one of 10,000 individual chemical reactions occurring each second in trillions of cells in your body requires a mineral to make it happen!

We are fortunate to work with a small company in the southeastern United States that has produced liquid minerals since the 1970s from a deposit of prehistoric vegetation, which has been composted over millions of years into "humic shale," or clay, rich in fulvic acid. On page 113, you'll find Miracles With Minerals, which describes some of the many healing uses for liquid minerals.

Not all liquid mineral products are equally potent, balanced, or effective, so buy carefully! Many popular brands are diluted so much that several ounces per day may be required, and some are not even from plant sources, which makes them useless internally. Those we use come from a plant deposit, and require a relatively small amount per day.

Putting It All Together

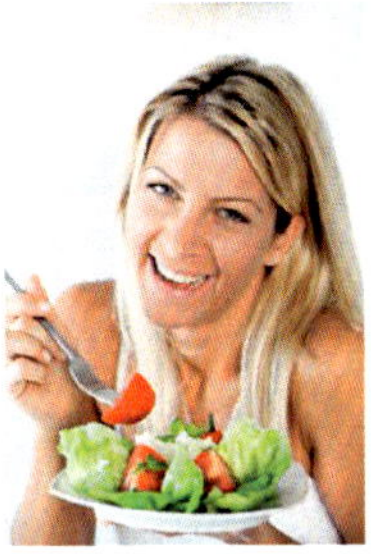

You should have your fridge stocked by now from the list of foods to eat, and you've eliminated the ones to avoid. You have nuts and seeds germinating, and you've mixed three *Cranberry-Vinegar-Lemon* drinks for the day. Now, you're ready to put everything together to make all the pieces fit.

REMEMBER: Eat plenty to be satisfied, including snacks between meals!

Sample Menus and Combinations

BREAKFASTS:

- Cut vegetables with raw nuts, plus an apple with almond butter
- Sautéed mushrooms and onions, plus raw nuts
- Fresh berries or other fruit with plain low-fat yogurt or cottage cheese
- Plain low-fat yogurt with applesauce
- Low-fat cottage cheese with pineapple chunks
- Low-fat yogurt topped with nuts or seeds
- Whole grapefruit

LUNCHES:

- Steamed or broiled asparagus with butter, sliced tomatoes and cucumbers, plus an apple with raw nuts or almond butter
- Steamed broccoli and bell peppers with butter, plus an apple with nuts or almond butter
- Salad with sliced almonds, plus an apple
- Mixed fruit salad plus sunflower or pumpkin seeds

DINNERS:

- Steamed or sautéed cauliflower with butter, plus a salad with almonds
- Cooked lima beans, plus a salad
- Steamed kale, radish greens, collards, beet greens and sliced beets, plus hummus and sliced carrots, peppers and celery
- Falafel balls or patties over salad
- Organic prepared mushroom soup with sliced mushrooms, onion, garlic and broccoli, plus crisp bread spread thinly with Boursin cheese and topped with sprouts
- Spaghetti squash with sliced black olives and sautéed mushrooms topped with marinara sauce

BETWEEN MEAL SNACKS:

- Carrot and celery sticks with almond butter or tahini
- Apple slices with almond butter or nuts

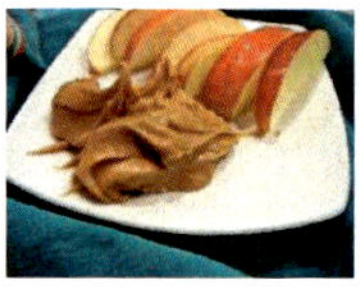

- Mixed raw nuts and seeds, with or without an apple
- Whole grapefruit or a bowl of fresh berries
- Hummus with apple slices
- Guacamole with assorted vegetable

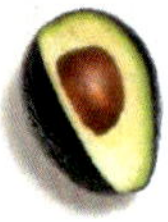

SALAD SUGGESTIONS:

Almost any vegetable mix can become an enormous salad that will last for days! Imagination is the only limit to the variety of vegetables (and even a few fruits) that can be combined to make fantastic salads.

GREENS:

- kale
- field greens
- romaine
- arugula
- baby spinach

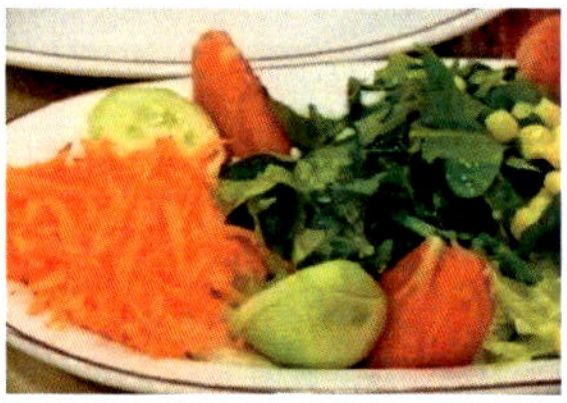

OTHER VEGETABLES:

- cucumbers
- celery
- shredded beets
- carrots
- red cabbage
- jicama
- broccoli
- cauliflower
- onion
- mushrooms
- radishes

SALAD TOPPINGS:

- tomato
- sprouts
- avocado
- nuts or seeds
- cooked peas, lentils, beans, or falafel
- pineapple chunks
- apple or pear chunks
- black or green olives
- artichoke hearts

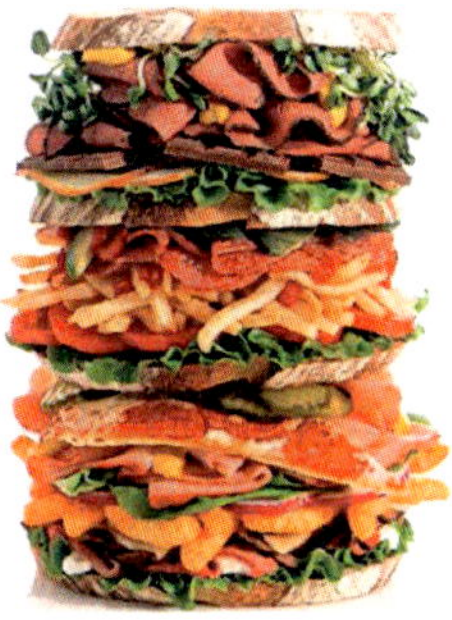

Why We Feel Hungry or Satisfied

Refined or "empty foods" act like stimulants. Breads and other processed carbohydrates trigger "hunger" signals in the brain. That's why you can eat a large amount of refined carbohydrates before feeling satisfied.

Eating complex carbohydrates, such as those found in raw vegetables, triggers "satisfied" signals in the brain's hunger centers. When the body gets the nutrition it needs, the result is less hunger and eventually cravings disappear.

What to Expect

With the liver's enhanced ability to utilize hormones, almost everyone notices improvement in hair, nails, skin and sex drive. Improved liver function will also help normalize blood pressure, blood sugar and cholesterol regulation. If you take medication, consult your doctor to adjust dosages as needed.

At the end of two weeks, you should notice that cravings are reduced or eliminated; bowel movements and energy level should be improved; weight and inches should be dropping off.

If you drop five pounds or less, your body is most likely re-building its lean body mass and needs more time to heal. Eating protein also slows down the elimination of excess weight.

Excess water will be eliminated before fat-burning kicks in. The maximum healthy pace of fat-weight elimination is about two pounds per week, when organs and hormones are working properly.

Your overall health will largely determine how much fat is eliminated and how quickly.

What Will You Do After the Two Weeks?

It will take more than two weeks to regenerate the liver fully; this is only the beginning! The liver is one of many organs involved in hormone regulation, digestion, detoxification, elimination, and other functions that are easily taken for granted.

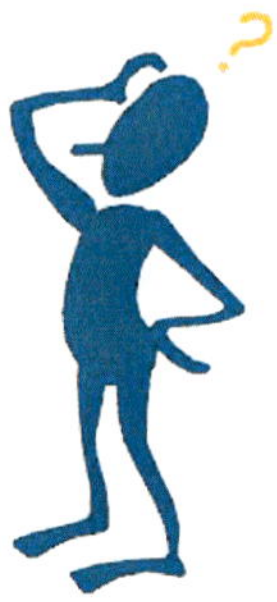

The goal is always restoring and sustaining optimal health and well-being. Some people continue this process for another one to three weeks, or even several months. If your results are good, it is perfectly safe to extend the program for as long as you wish.

One client, who saw vast improvements in blood pressure, sleep and mood, began modifying the program to allow some of his former eating habits to creep back in. It didn't take long for him to notice that his progress came to a screeching halt.

When he resumed observing the guidelines, his body started to cleanse, rebuild and heal. He regained the improvements he had made previously and dropped more weight. He was eventually able to reintroduce some of his favorite foods, not as daily habits, but as occasional treats.

Eat only food that will spoil (before it spoils)**.**

Eat only food made by God.

"God food, not lab food."

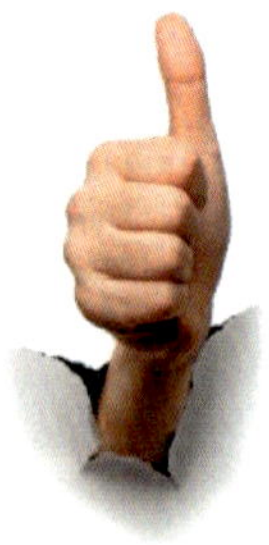

The process above was adapted, in part, from the book, *Healthy Hormones, Healthy Life*, by Eric Berg, D.C.

THE ROYAL FLUSH®

THE SAFEST, MOST EFFECTIVE INTESTINAL CLEANSE YOU'LL EVER USE

The ROYAL FLUSH®, when used to replace one meal per day, is a superior, safe, easy, and effective method of cleansing years of built-up waste in the intestinal tract, and ridding the body of accumulated toxins. Many methods of colon cleansing are available and some are more effective than others. They may include pills, capsules, powders, suppositories, candies, chewing gum, drinks, enemas or colonics, and even surgical procedures.

According to experts in the field of natural health, many chronic health problems have their origin in poor dietary habits, faulty digestion, lack of efficient nutrient absorption, and poor elimination of waste.

Elie Metchnikoff, the Nobel prize-winning Russian biologist, is credited with the statement, *"Death begins in the colon,"* which is often evidenced by a host of symptoms, some of which are so slight as to go unnoticed or be taken for granted as part of normal aging processes.

"Leaky Gut Syndrome" is a common diagnosis given to those with symptoms of toxic build-up in the colon.

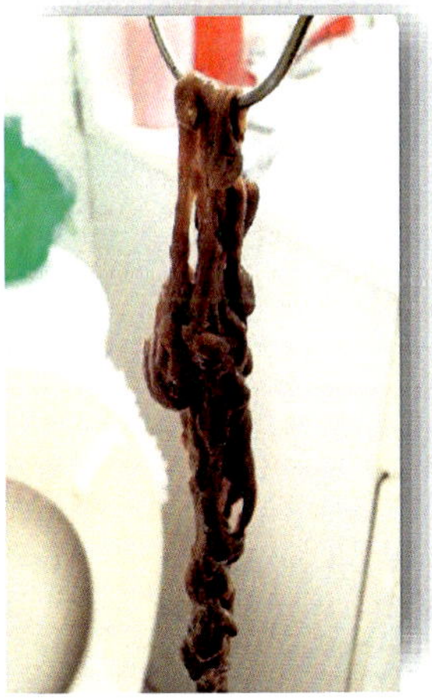

You may find it hard to believe that built-up waste like this picture could be in your intestines, but the proof is in the toilet! If you've eaten white flour, white sugar, fried, processed or fast foods, or have not had proper elimination (2 to 3 times a day), you would benefit from the ROYAL FLUSH®!

Most people enjoy a decrease in food cravings, stabilized appetite, increased energy, improved memory, and elimination of excess fat and weight. They may be preventing other health problems too!

Residue of built-up waste in the intestines may become hardened, creating a "pipe" around the lining of the tissue walls, which prevents efficient assimilation of nutrients needed for optimum health. Venus Andrecht, author of *The Herb Lady's Notebook*, interviewed nurses who assisted surgeries during which colons had to be removed with a hacksaw!

Some people may have malformed colons with kinks, bulges, balloons or collapsed areas and others may also have restrictions due to accidents or surgery. Obstructions can also occur in the small intestines.

All of these areas are potential problems since waste accumulation allows toxins to be continually and easily released into the blood stream and recycled through the entire body.

Normal bowel movements should occur two to three times per day. If this is not the case, consider performing the simple and effective **SALTWATER FLUSH** on page 53 as a way of encouraging normal bowel movement. You may also benefit from using the herb, *cascara sagrada*, to increase the wave-like peristaltic action of the colon.

Commercial products to assist bowel movement and regularity, and the amount needed, will vary from individual to individual. If you choose such a preparation, start by using the directions on the label, and increase or decrease the amounts slowly to achieve the desired results.

If you are accustomed to infrequent bowel movements, it may take several weeks to establish proper colon activity.

Before beginning the ROYAL FLUSH®, be certain that your bowels are moving *at least* once a day without help for a week.

INGREDIENTS FOR THE ROYAL FLUSH®

- **LIQUID DETOX CLAY**

All natural Bentonite, (volcanic clay) works like a magnet to attract toxic substances, clean out mucus, and assist in their removal. **DETOX CLAY** is no longer available, but **SONNE'S #7** (available online) is an equally powerful detoxifying agent, binding up to 40 times its weight in toxins, and helping rid the body of harmful bacteria and parasites.

- **CLEAN SWEEP MIX™**

Mixed with **ALKALINE IONIZED WATER** or reverse osmosis (RO) water and apple juice (with or without whole-leaf Aloe Vera juice), works as a broom to clean and nourish the colon. (Recipe on p. 36)

- **APPLE JUICE**

Organic, unfiltered apple juice contains carbohydrates that satisfy, burn slowly, and offer a great source of energy. The next best choice is organic bottled juice. Whole-leaf aloe vera juice may be substituted if allergies, blood sugar problems, or Candida (yeast) prohibit the use of apple juice.

- **TRACE MINERALS PLUS+®**

The key to the **ROYAL FLUSH**®, this unique solution of macro and trace minerals cleans off the colon lining like a chisel and kills parasites, while it heals the delicate tissues at the same time. No other minerals work as well; *we know because we've tried others!*

- **PROBIOTICS** (optional)

Healthy bacteria, such as *Acidophilus* and *Bifidus*, help re-establish a proper intestinal environment, as waste and toxins are flushed out. Probiotics should be taken at least 30 minutes before a meal, or two hours after meals, to ensure that the beneficial bacteria are not denatured in the stomach before they reach the intestinal tract.

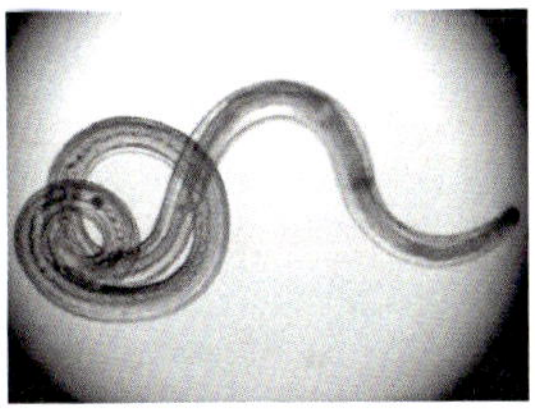

Many people eliminate parasites while on the **ROYAL FLUSH**®, in addition to tumors, and unidentifiable masses of varying shapes, colors and sizes. The proof is in the toilet!

ROYAL FLUSH® RECIPE

FIRST: On an empty stomach, take 1 tablespoon SONNE'S #7 (DETOX CLAY)

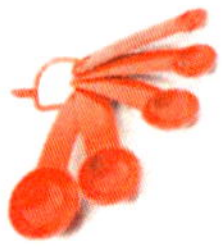

- **3 hours before flush** (2 hours works, but 3 is better).
- **Use a plastic measuring spoon** – ***NEVER*** let it touch metal!
- **Rinse your mouth** after swallowing, and sip a little water.

SECOND: Mix in your BLENDERBOTTLE® (2-3 hours after SONNE'S #7)

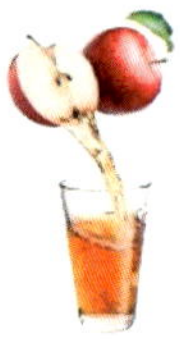

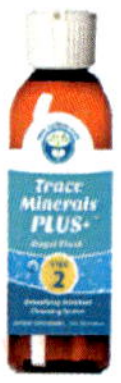

- **12 oz. organic apple juice -** Unfiltered if possible.
  (Use whole leaf aloe vera juice for Candida or blood sugar problems)
- **12 oz.** ALKALINE IONIZED, reverse osmosis, or filtered water
- **1 teaspoon*** **of** TRACE MINERALS PLUS+®
- **3 LEVEL Tablespoons*** **of** CLEAN SWEEP MIX™ – Recipe:
  - 21 oz (600 grams) of organic psyllium husk powder
  - 7 oz (200 grams) of organic whole psyllium husk
  - 3.5 oz (100 grams) of organic green power blend

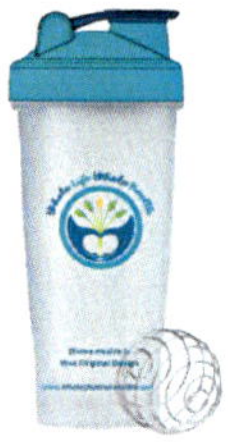

* Use only ½ amounts for the first three to four days.

THIRD: Shake well and drink fast! (The fiber in CLEAN SWEEP MIX™ swells quickly.) Wait 2-3 hours to eat.

Continue the **ROYAL FLUSH®** until *all* abnormal, rubber-like, hardened, mucus-like toxins are eliminated. Continue for an additional two weeks, then stay off for two weeks, and then try the flush again to see if any more abnormal toxins are eliminated. If not, repeat the **ROYAL FLUSH®** once a week or at least once a month, depending on your diet.

Your first **ROYAL FLUSH®** "adventure" may take a few weeks to a few months to complete.

> **Brush your teeth after drinking the ROYAL FLUSH®, so TRACE MINERALS PLUS+® won't stain your teeth!**

The Process

Replace one meal every day with the Royal Flush® (no food for 2-3 hours before, during or after). Replacing breakfast is a popular practice, although some people find it easier to replace lunch or dinner. Whatever meal you choose to replace, drink *all* of the **Royal Flush®**. Remember that the "broom" (Clean Sweep Mix™) needs volume to "push" it.

It is normal to experience varying degrees of abdominal bloating and distention. Depending on the level of toxicity in your body, mild headaches or slight, flu-like symptoms may occur. Before being completely eliminated, toxins will be released into the blood stream after being loosened from the intestinal walls. To eliminate unpleasant symptoms, use only half the recipe for the first three to four days, and then increase to the full recipe.

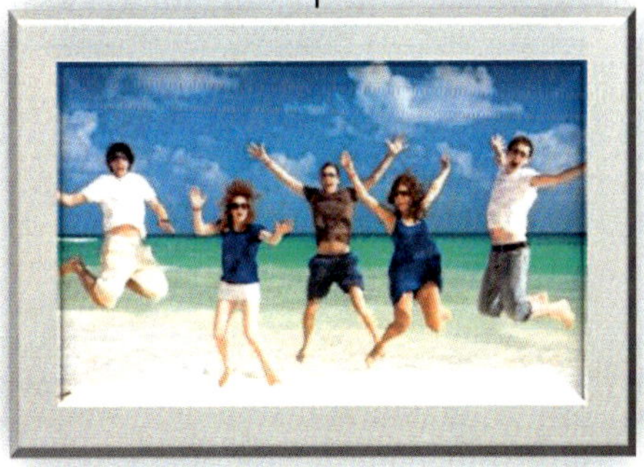

Continue the Royal Flush® until the stool looks normal for at least 7 consecutive days. The duration of this cleanse is determined by the extent of accumulated waste. An adult who has never cleansed his or her colon should plan to be on the **Royal Flush®** for at least three months, or until the desired results are reached.

The Proof is in the Toilet!

When you find black, rubbery, hardened, rope-like, mucous-laden material in the stool, you'll know your intestines are cleaning out!

Other cleansing regimens that you may want to consider, along with the **Royal Flush®** include the 2-week **Liver Rejuvenating Program**, followed by the **4-Day Kidney, Liver, Gallbladder Cleanse**.

TIPS FOR THE ROYAL FLUSH®

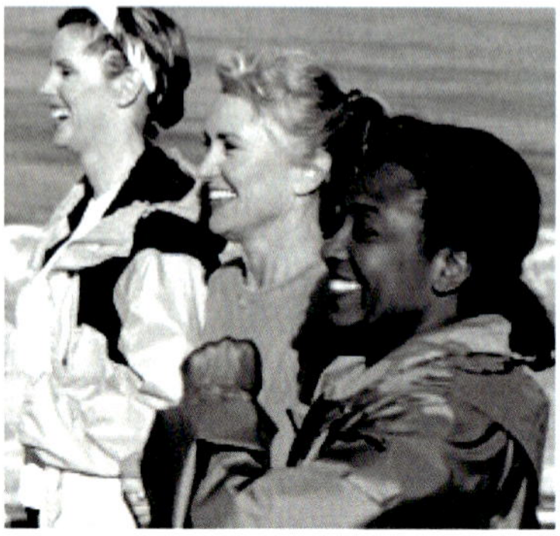

- Add a few drops of liquid Stevia extract if desired to help the **ROYAL FLUSH®** drink taste better.
- CLEAN SWEEP MIX™ has proven to be the most effective blend of soluble and insoluble fiber by far, without being harsh.
- **Probiotics may be taken during the ROYAL FLUSH®** to support healthy bacterial flora in the intestines.
- **You may need help to eliminate rubbery waste.** An already clogged colon requires an extra "push." See the **SALTWATER FLUSH** on page 53. Work with a holistic practitioner to determine what works best for you. Avoid prescription drugs if at all possible.
- **There may be bloating and gas during the first three or four days.** To reduce or eliminate burping, gas and bloating, use VEGETARIAN ENZYME COMPLEX with meals and snacks, and DAILY ENZYME COMPLEX between meals.
- **To maintain detoxification,** eat lots of vegetables, and *very little* animal protein.

KIDNEY, LIVER AND GALLBLADDER CLEANSES

The kidneys are your body's main blood-filtering organs. Their internal membranes, called *glomeruli*, are very delicate, and cleansing them properly is essential to any toxin removal program.

Any type of cleanse will be more effective and tolerated better if the organs responsible for handling the toxins are functioning properly.

Kidney stones can cause excruciating pain, and gallstones can cause symptoms that often result in thousands of preventable surgeries each year.

It is recommended that these cleanses be repeated at reasonable intervals (every two to three months) until stones and other waste materials have been cleared; and annually after that.

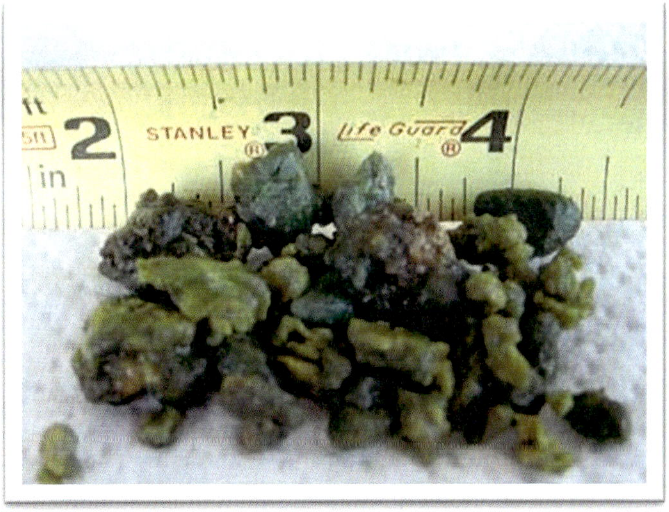

A photo of actual gallstones from a "*healthy*" gallbladder!

The "owner" had no symptoms and the stones passed painlessly.

3-Day Kidney Cleanse

Every day, for three days, drink ONLY apple juice and water (no other food or drink). Drink all you want, up to a gallon of each per day. You can mix the water and juice, or drink them separately. We have found it most effective to mix ½ apple juice and ½ water.

You will need three gallons of apple juice and three gallons of water. Look for unsweetened, unfiltered organic juice. Fresh, non-pasteurized cider (available directly from some orchards) is even better.

You won't starve! The mix is surprisingly satisfying, because the carbohydrates in apple juice burn slowly and offer a great source of energy. If you really must eat something, have an occasional apple, but try to keep this to a minimum.

After you first begin drinking apple juice and water, you can strain your urine to check for kidney stones. An ordinary mesh strainer works fine. The stones may be tiny, so look carefully.

Apple juice softens kidney stones, so they pass *painlessly!*

Use the Saltwater Flush each morning during these three days to help release toxins.

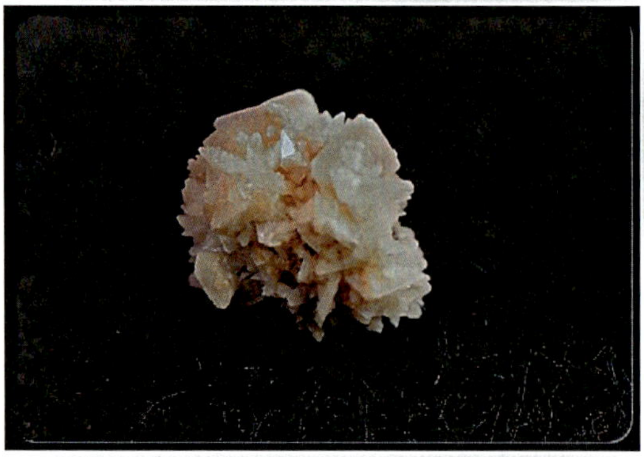

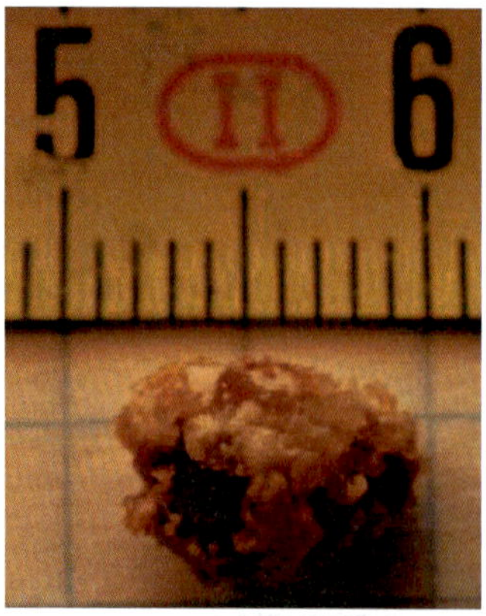

4-Day Kidney, Liver and Gallbladder Cleanse

For the first three days, follow the kidney cleanse with only apple juice and water. The liver and gallbladder cleanse actually starts on the third night of the kidney cleanse.

On the third day, be sure to have these on hand:

- 1/2 cup cold pressed extra-virgin olive oil, chilled
- 1/4 cup fresh-squeezed lemon juice

When you are completely ready for bed, drink the olive oil and lemon juice mixed together. It may be easier to drink through a straw to avoid tasting the oil.

After drinking the oil and lemon juice, you may feel like burping or even vomiting. If so, **a *sip* of tomato juice may help, but do not drink more than a tablespoon. Brush your teeth.**

Go directly to bed and lie on your *right* side, 4-5 hours, with two pillows under your hip. This may feel awkward, but it is the most effective position for expelling gallstones.

Sometime during the night you may feel nauseated or vomit. Do not be alarmed. This is caused by the gallbladder ejecting the stones with such force that oil shoots back into the stomach.

You may be able to feel the expulsion of gallstones. It won't be painful, but may feel like a mild contraction.

You may spend an uncomfortable night, *but it's only one night!* Remember, you're helping an important organ to work properly. You may also be avoiding gallbladder surgery, and future stress on the liver that cannot be undone!

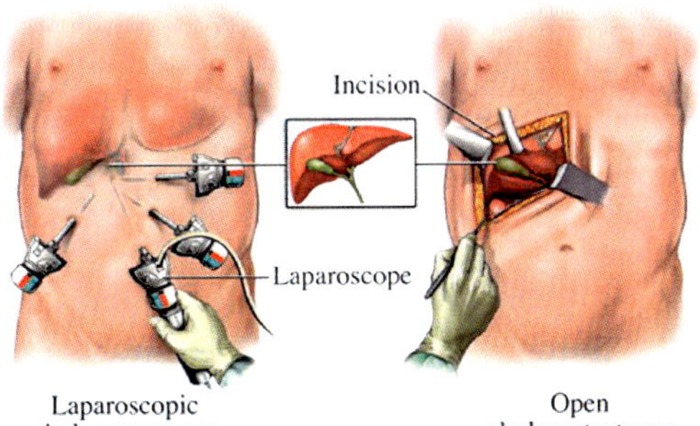

Laparoscopic cholecystectomy

Open cholecystectomy

Don't let this happen to you!

Continue drinking apple juice and water during the fourth day. Be prepared to spend the day resting, if necessary.

Sometime during the day you should have a bowel movement, during which gallstones will be eliminated. You may wish to apply ointment (like *Neem salve*) to the rectum before the bowel movement. This prevents any burning from toxins which may also be released with the stones.

When you pass gallstones, they will float on the water, because they are cholesterol-based. You will not feel pain when they pass, because they are soft and oily at this point.

It is not unusual to pass several dozen gallstones after doing this cleanse! Gallstones can be the size of peas or as large as the end of your thumb! The stones will be different shades of green to black. Light-colored stones are the newest; blackish stones are the oldest. The color comes from the bile.

It is rewarding to see the stones outside of your body, where they can do no more harm!

Gallstones break down after a few days, so, if you want to save your "treasures" and amaze your friends, be sure to freeze them!

Not everyone passes actual stones, but nearly everyone passes "chaff." This waste product is fibrous or scaly in texture and will float. Whether you produce chaff or stones, you should consider repeating the cleanse no sooner than two weeks.

Use the **SALTWATER FLUSH** each morning, on the fifth and sixth days, to help clean out any toxins remaining from the cleanse.

Eat sparingly on the fifth day, beginning with fresh vegetable juices and broths, gradually adding solid fruit and vegetables. Eat small meals and eat slowly.

Your body will have slowed down its digestive process, since no solid food was being eaten for four days, and it may take another three to four days to return to a normal diet. If you experience any discomfort after eating, introduce foods more gradually.

24-Hour Liver Cleanse

- 2:00 pm: **Stop all food and liquids.** Sip only a little water if you are very thirsty.
- 6:00 pm: **Drink 3/4 cup water mixed with 1 Tablespoon Epsom salts.** You may add a few drops of lemon juice to improve the taste.

  NOTE: Epsom salts may cause abdominal cramps for a few hours, due to gas.
- 8:00 pm: **Repeat the water and Epsom salts.**
- 9:45 pm: **Mix thoroughly 1/2 cup cold-pressed olive oil with 3/4 cup fresh-squeezed grapefruit juice** and drink the mixture.
- **Go directly to bed** and lie on your right side, with your right leg drawn up.
- **Upon waking** (anytime after 6:00 am), **take a third dose of Epsom salts and water. Expect diarrhea in the morning.**
- **After two hours, take your fourth** – and last – **dose of Epsom salts and water.**
- **After two more hours, you may start to eat.** Proceed slowly – start with fruit. You might want to plan for a light day.

Completing the **3-Day Kidney Cleanse** is recommended before starting this process.

21-Day Gradual Cleanse

This diet will gradually clear the liver and gallbladder. During this process, **avoid foods rich in saturated fats** (red meat, dairy, eggs, etc.). **Also avoid peanuts, nuts and seeds.**

- **Eat primarily vegetables, fruit, unrefined grains and legumes.** Pears, parsnips, seaweed, lemons, limes, and the spice, turmeric, will hasten gallstone removal and should be emphasized in the diet.
- **Eat two radishes a day between meals.** Radishes help remove deposits from the gallbladder and liver.
- **Drink 3 to 5 cups of tea each day,** either 3 cups of cleavers tea (gallium aparine), or 5 cups of chamomile tea (anthernis nobilis).
- **Pour 5 teaspoons of fresh, cold-pressed flaxseed oil over food** at one meal each day, or take the equivalent in encapsulated oil. **Continue using flaxseed oil in this manner for at least two months.**

Posted on mercola.com in 2002

Obviously, this is a much slower cleanse than the ones previously discussed. The specific foods and herbs are usually sufficient to remove stones and chaff from the liver and gallbladder over a period of three weeks. The process may be extended to a few months, depending on how congested the liver and gallbladder are.

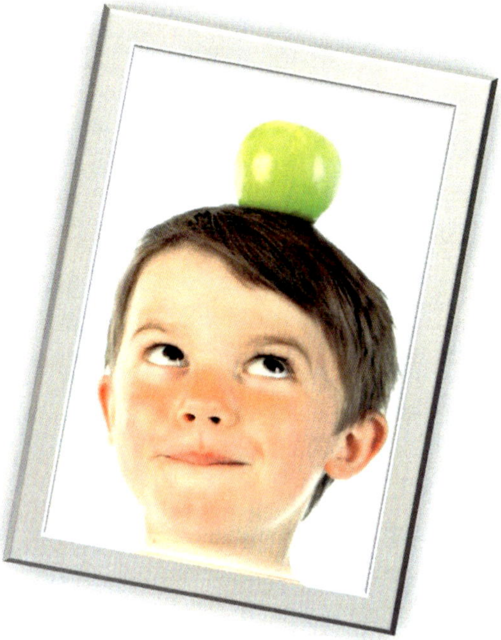

24-Hour Apple Lover's Cleanse

- EAT ONLY APPLES* throughout the day, preferably organic. Eat as many as desired, but at least four to five.

***Green apples seem to work best.**

- DRINK WATER, **herbal teas, and/or apple juice.**

- AT BEDTIME, **mix 1/3 cup fresh-squeezed lemon juice with 2/3 cup cold-pressed extra virgin olive oil.** Drink the mixture and then go immediately to bed, lying on your right side, with your right leg drawn up.

Stones and/or chaff should pass in the stool the next morning.

3-Month Mild Flush

1. **For five consecutive days**, drink the following mixture on an empty stomach:

    - 2 tablespoons of cold-pressed extra virgin olive oil
    - 2 tablespoons of freshly squeezed lemon juice

2. **Skip the next five days**.

3. **Repeat steps one and two above** for at least three months.

Fruit Pectin Liver Detox

Pectin is a water-soluble fiber found in most fruit, which shows an ability to bind with cholesterol. This property makes pectin a valuable supplement for assisting liver and gallbladder detoxification. Instead of drinking large amounts of fruit juice, or eating large quantities of whole fruit, using only pectin helps avoid increasing blood sugar, which may be challenging for some people.

1. **Add one packet of pectin* to one quart of water and stir vigorously.** *We recommend the Ball Fruit Jell brand.
2. **Drink three 4-ounce glasses of this solution per day** for at least one month, or follow your holistic practitioner's instructions.

TIPS FOR KIDNEY, LIVER AND GALLBLADDER CLEANSES

✓ JUICE QUALITY MATTERS

Fresh juice from organically grown fruit is always best. Bottled lemon or grapefruit juice will not produce good results. When it comes to cranberry juice, look for organic, unfiltered, unsweetened juice. When cranberries are over-cooked, or if refined sugars or corn sweeteners are added, the juice becomes acid-producing and should be avoided.

✓ NAUSEA OR HEADACHES

Your body may release toxins faster than it can eliminate them. DETOX CLAY absorbs many of these toxins, making it easier for your system to tolerate the cleansing process. **DETOX CLAY** is available as SONNE'S #7 online. Follow the instructions on the label.

✓ OLIVE OIL

Chilling olive oil can make it more tolerable to drink.

✓ DRINKING THE OIL

Drink the oil and lemon juice mixture through a straw, at the back of the mouth to help avoid any unpleasant taste. Then brush your teeth.

✓ CONSTIPATION

If this becomes a problem, use one of the products already discussed. Also refer to the **SALTWATER FLUSH** on page 53.

✓ DIARRHEA

Loose stools and even some diarrhea may result from either the **4-DAY KIDNEY, LIVER AND GALL-BLADDER CLEANSE** or the **24-HOUR LIVER CLEANSE**. This should be temporary, and normal stool should return within a day or so of resuming solid food.

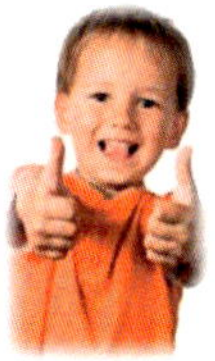

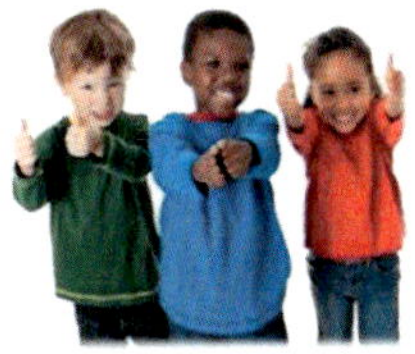

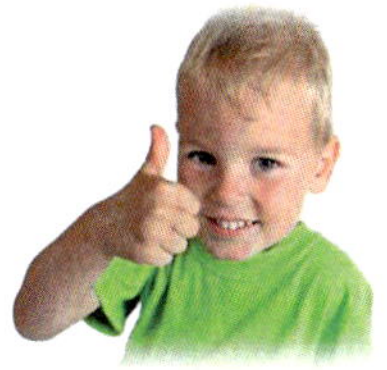

Whole-Body Cellular Cleanse

Cellular cleanses are designed to accomplish the following:

- Dissolve and eliminate toxins and congestion that have formed in any part of the body
- Eliminate unusable wastes which accumulate in joints and muscles
- Purify the entire body
- Relieve irritation and inflammation in the nerves, arteries and blood vessels
- Regain skin elasticity
- Improve energy levels
- Flush mucus build-up
- Dissolve fat

"I went on my first 40-day cleansing fast at 57 years old!"

1. First, I did the **4-Day Kidney, Liver and Gallbladder Cleanse**
2. From the 5th to the 40th day, I did the **Lemonade Cleanse**
3. During the entire 40 days, I was also doing the **Royal Flush®** to cleanse the toxins from my colon, and to keep things moving.

"The 40 days were a wonderful time of rejuvenation and renewal. I felt great, had lots of energy and a sense of lightness. I continued my exercise program and all of my usual daily activities. I also entered into this as a spiritual fast. As Jesus said, ***'This cannot be driven out by anything but prayer and fasting'*** (Mark 9:29, AMP). I figured I'd do my part and God would do His. It worked, Praise the Lord!" *Barbara Brown, MSE*

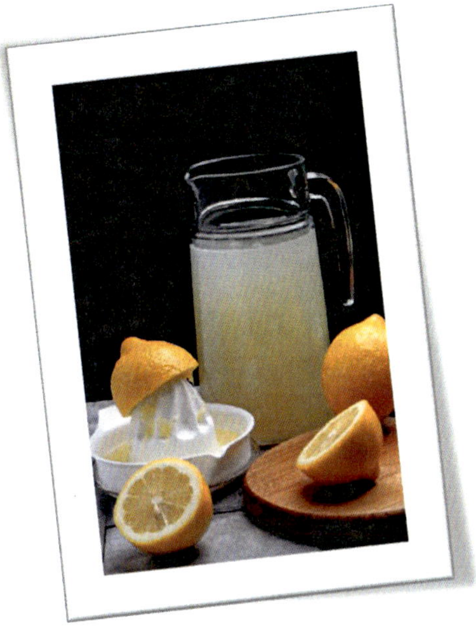

10-Day Lemonade Cellular Cleanse

This is one of the most effective cellular cleanses we've ever found. The cleansing properties of fresh lemon (or lime) juice are astonishing, and have resulted in the almost miraculous elimination of ulcers, allergies, joint pain and stiffness, skin problems (fungus, acne, etc.), respiratory conditions, and other health threats.

It may seem hard to believe that sufficient nutrition could be contained in so simple a formula, but the **Lemonade Cellular Cleanse** supplies the essential nutrients for 10 to 40 days, and may even be repeated three to four times in a single year.

The lemonade formula has tremendous capacity to dissolve fatty tissue, mineral deposits in joints and muscles, and clean mucus membranes. Elimination of stubborn weight is also a benefit.

Cholesterol levels may be lowered during even a 10-Day Lemonade Cellular Cleanse.

The Lemonade Cleanse

MAY BE USED SEVERAL DIFFERENT WAYS

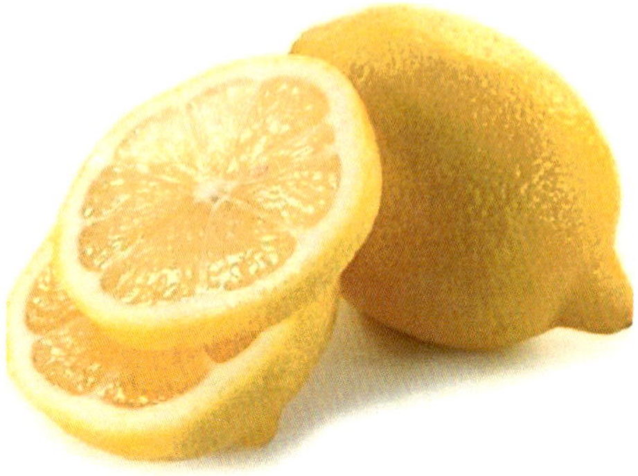

AS A FAST: For a period of 10 to 40 days, consume only the lemonade (drink at least 6-12 glasses per day).

AS A DAILY REGIMEN: Consume only the lemonade and water until 4 p.m.; then eat a healthy, balanced dinner, with fruit for dessert, if desired.

AS A TONIC: Drink one glass of lemonade first thing in the morning and just before bed in the evening.

Recipe

- **2 Tablespoons fresh squeezed lemon or lime juice**
- **2 Tablespoons pure maple syrup** (Dark or Very Dark)
- **1/10 teaspoon cayenne pepper**
- **10 ounces water**

Ingredients

LEMON OR LIME JUICE – *Fresh organic fruit is best.* Lemons and limes are among the richest sources of minerals and vitamins of any food known to man and are mucous-dissolving. Even though they are acidic fruits, they become alkaline as they are digested and assimilated.

Never vary the amount of juice per glass and never use canned or bottled juice.

MAPLE SYRUP – *Use only real maple syrup.* Grade A Dark or Very Dark is less refined and contains more nutrients. Maple syrup has a wide variety of minerals and vitamins such as iron, calcium and magnesium, Vitamins A, B1, B2, B6, and C. For those who are overweight, less maple syrup may be taken, or more may be added for those who are underweight.

CAYENNE PEPPER – *Start cautiously with cayenne pepper* and work up to as much as you can tolerate. We recommend adding cayenne to each glassful of lemonade just before you drink it rather than putting a large amount in a pitcher of lemonade.

> Powdered cayenne seems to gain heat the longer it sits in liquid. A liquid cayenne tincture is available and seems to be easier to use, as it can be added to the lemonade at any time.

Cayenne pepper helps break up mucus, cleanses bronchial tubes and sinus cavities, increases and strengthens the blood supply, and may even help soothe ulcers and stop hemorrhages.

ADAPTING FOR DIABETES: Substitute *blackstrap molasses* for maple syrup, beginning with no more than a level tablespoon per glass during the first day. The amount of molasses may be increased up to two tablespoons per glass. Then, *slowly* begin replacing the molasses with maple syrup until it is tolerated well. *Monitor blood sugar often and adjust insulin levels as needed.*

> **Don't be surprised if your insulin requirement is greatly reduced or even eliminated!**

If you have been diagnosed with diabetes, work closely with your physician or holistic practitioner during this process, and keep them informed of your progress.

LEMONADE RECIPE BY THE PITCHER

- **¾ cup fresh squeezed lemon or lime juice**
- **¾ cup pure maple syrup** (Dark or Very Dark)
- **8 cups water**
- **Add 1/10 tsp. cayenne pepper to each 10 oz. glass**

The Lemonade Cleanse was originally published as the Master Cleanse by Stanley Burroughs.

Coming off the Lemonade Cleanse

- **FIRST DAY:** Drink several 8-ounce glasses of fresh orange juice as desired, which prepares the digestive system to assimilate food properly.
- **SECOND DAY:** Drink several 8-ounce glasses of fresh orange juice. In the afternoon and evening, eat some fresh vegetable soup.
- **THIRD DAY:** Drink orange juice in the morning. At noon, have some fresh vegetable soup. In the evening, eat whatever fruit or vegetables are desired. Grains, dairy products and meats should be added *slowly* and *sparingly*.

Congratulations! You did it!

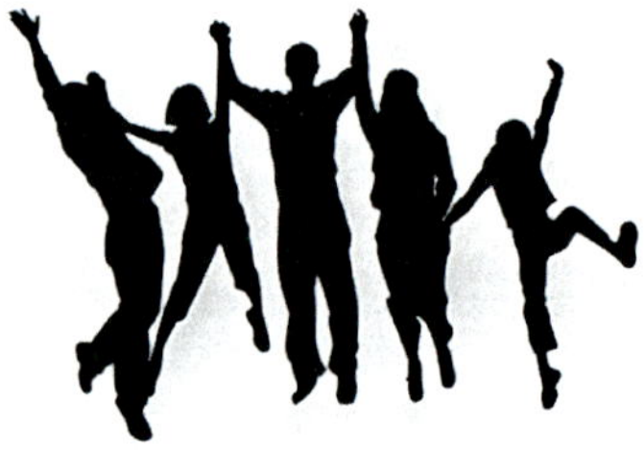

What to Expect From a Cellular Cleanse

It is important to refrain from eating refined sugars or grains while on this or any cleanse. This avoids creating spikes in blood sugar levels that cause unnecessary hunger and cravings.

In the early stages of detoxification, some people experience a reaction to the toxins that are being released into the system. Headaches, nausea, dizziness, and joint pain, or weakness can be eased by taking one or two tablespoons of liquid Bentonite, or Detox Clay (Sonne's #7), with lots of water.

If you experience severe symptoms, or if symptoms persist longer than a few days, consult your holistic practitioner for assistance.

After a few days you should be energized and feeling great! This is a perfect time to begin a new food lifestyle!

Special Cleanses

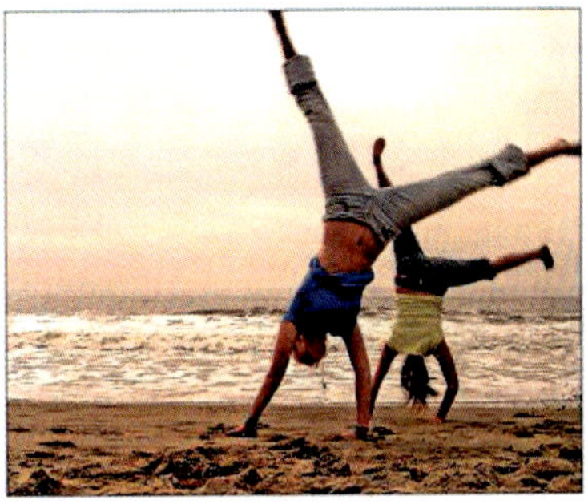

The Saltwater Flush

Salt has been used throughout the ages to draw out poisons and as an anti-bacterial agent. The **Saltwater Flush** provides an internal bath, flushing toxins without the harmful effects of chemical laxatives. Unlike colonics or enemas, which can only reach into the large intestine, or a small part of it, the **Saltwater Flush** removes toxins as it cleanses the *entire* digestive tract.

Salt will do no harm when used in this way, and will sterilize, making it easier for the body to repair the tissues.

Saltwater Recipe

- **2 level teaspoons of unrefined sea salt.** *(Do not use ordinary iodized salt.)*
- **1 quart warm water.**
- **Mix in a 1-quart container.** Shake or stir well to dissolve completely.
- **Drink the entire quart of saltwater** first thing in the morning. It must be taken on an empty stomach. *Using a straw can make it easier to drink the mixture.*

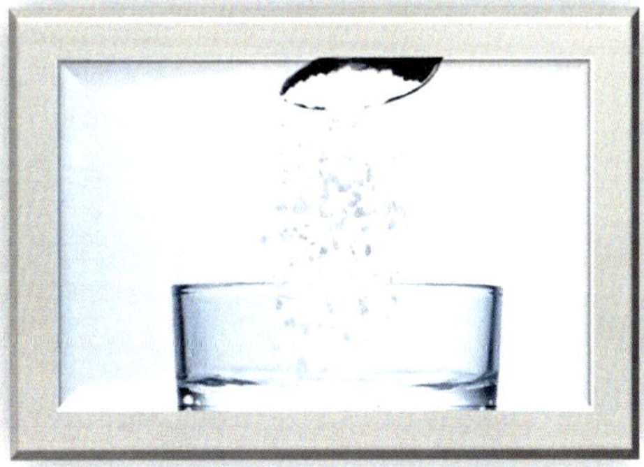

- **Lie on your right side for 30 minutes** after drinking the saltwater.

Tips for the Saltwater Flush

- The saltwater mixture will not be absorbed and will stay intact to wash the entire digestive tract thoroughly in just a few hours.
- Most people will have bowel elimination in 1 to 2 hours.
  - ✓ **Multiple eliminations are common.**
- **Be careful passing gas:** Liquid will be coming through your system.
- The **Saltwater Flush** can be used daily if needed.
- **If constipation has been a chronic problem**, it may be advisable to take an herbal laxative tea at night, or use the herb, *cascara sagrada*, to loosen fecal matter and then drink the **Saltwater Flush** the next morning.

Urinary Tract and Bladder Cleanse

Urinary tract infections are often characterized by frequent, painful urination. The urine itself may have a strong odor and may appear cloudy. Symptoms may also include back pain, lower abdominal pain and pressure, and even fever as the body tries to throw off the infection.

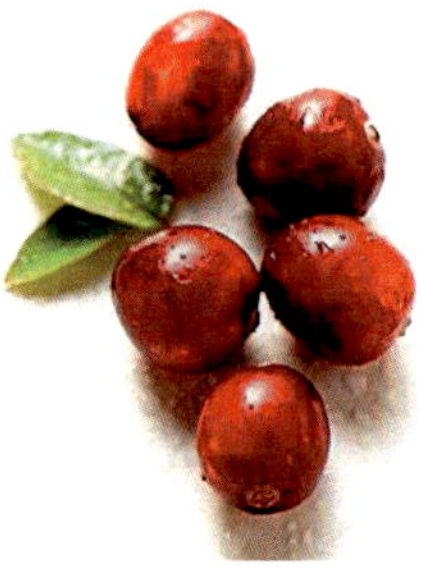

Cranberry juice has been used for many years as a natural remedy for urinary tract and bladder infections. Studies have shown that the beneficial effects of cranberries are real and complex. For example, bacteria must be able to adhere to the walls of the bladder before they can reproduce. A colony may then form which invades deeper into the tissue, causing inflammation. Laboratory studies have revealed that cranberry juice contains certain water-soluble compounds, which drastically reduce the ability of bacteria to adhere to the walls of the bladder. These special compounds bind to the bacteria, "confusing" them and effectively blocking their attachment. The bacteria are quickly washed from the bladder during urination.

Three Steps to Cleanse the Urinary Tract and Bladder

1. **Drink at least one quart of pure cranberry juice each day.**
2. **Drink 8 ounces of water every hour to keep wastes flushed.**
3. **Cleanse the urinary tract for at least 48 hours past the time you feel symptoms.**

As soon as pain or a burning sensation is noticed when urinating, begin drinking cranberry juice. The sooner you start, the less chance bacteria have to gain a foothold.

Freshly squeezed juice from organically grown fruit is always best. Look for unsweetened, unfiltered, organic cranberry juice.

Eat lightly during this cleanse

Eat foods with high water content such as fresh fruit and vegetables during this cleanse, but avoid oranges and grapefruit.

AVOID THESE:

- Coffee
- Chocolate
- Carbonated beverages
- Black tea
- Tomatoes
- Cooked spinach
- Yeasted breads
- Fried and fatty foods
- Sugar
- Salt
- Dairy foods
- Refined foods

Thanks to Dr. Marianne Hoyle, who contributed information for the preceding cleanses.
Also, thanks to Embassy of Heaven for the booklet *"Cleansing or Surgery."*

Oil Pulling
Not a "Cleanse," Yet it Cleanses

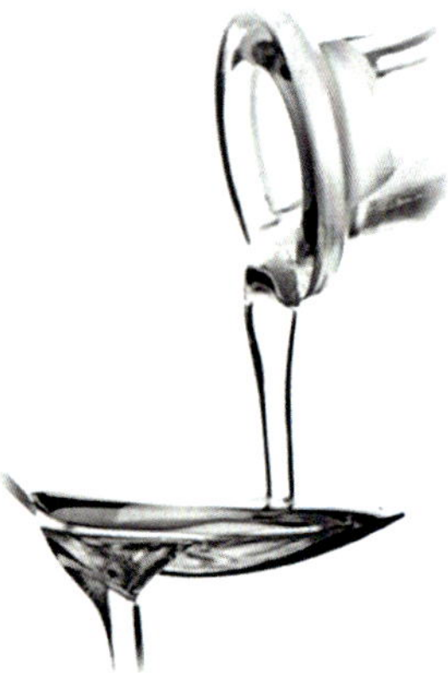

Friends in Nashville, Tennessee told us about the ancient Ayurvedic practice of **Oil Pulling** a few years ago. They had used the process to heal issues with their teeth and gums, and the results enabled them to avoid extensive and costly dental work. Obviously, we were impressed and when we faced oral health issues, we tried the practice ourselves with great success, and we have since recommended **Oil Pulling** enthusiastically.

Oil Pulling is the simple process of swishing around a tablespoon of sesame or sunflower oil in the mouth for about 20 minutes, thereby "pulling" it through the teeth, around the gums, and thoroughly bathing the inside of the mouth.

Here's how we do it . . .

YOU'LL NEED THREE ITEMS:

1. Bottle of sesame or sunflower oil
2. Tablespoon
3. Hydrogen Peroxide
   (mix half-and-half with purified water)

THE PROCESS:

1. Perform first thing upon waking
2. Take 1 tablespoon of oil in the mouth
3. Swish it around for 15-20 minutes
4. Spit out the oil in toilet (don't swallow it)
5. Rinse and gargle with the peroxide mix
6. Brush your teeth and start your day

THAT'S IT!

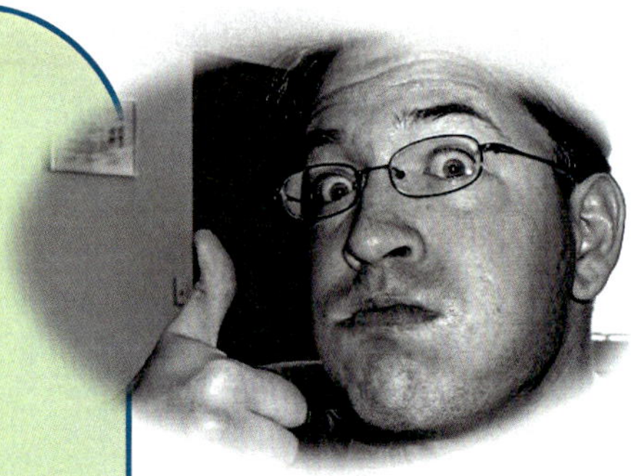

Find more information at mercola.com

ARE YOU ACID OR ALKALINE?
THE MAGIC OF pH

The single most important thing you can do to restore and sustain optimal health and well-being is establish and maintain an alkaline body chemistry.

All of the cleanses discussed in this book help to promote an alkaline body chemistry. The importance of this is impossible to overemphasize.

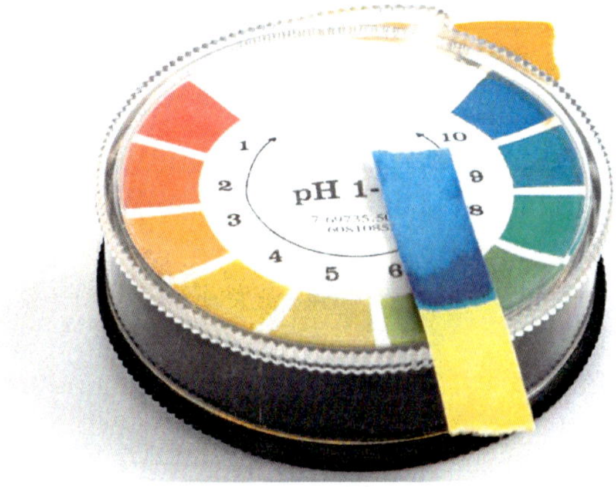

Dr. Otto Heinrich Warburg was awarded the Nobel Prize in 1931 for discovering the cause of cancer eight years earlier. What Dr. Warburg discovered is profound:

> ***"Cancerous cells can live and develop even in the absence of oxygen."***
> [i.e., in an acidic environment]
> Otto Heinrich Warburg, MD, Nobel Laureate

Dr. Warburg illustrated how changing the internal body chemistry from acidic to alkaline makes it impossible for cancer cells to live, and provides an environment in which healthy cells thrive.

Checking your pH gives you a picture of your TRUE health status.

URINE pH shows how good your diet *really* is. **Check every 3 months**

SALIVA pH shows how well you're handling stress. **Check every 2 weeks**

WHAT IS pH?

The measurement, known as pH, stands for *"potential of Hydrogen."* For our purposes, however, you can consider it as your *"personal health indicator."* The pH scale measures relative acidity or alkalinity using numbers ranging from 1 to 14.

You can see on the chart below that less than 7.0 is acidic and more than 7.0 is alkaline. Vinegar, for example, would measure around 2.5, while ammonia might measure 12.0.

ACID IS FOR BATTERIES, NOT BODIES.

Your insides are alkaline by design, and create acid, called *carbonic acid*, as a byproduct of metabolism – the process of simply being alive – and you breathe most of it out as carbon dioxide.

The ideal blood pH is 7.4, to carry maximum oxygen to all of your cells, and your body works hard to keep blood pH in a very narrow range (7.35-7.45).

pH SCALE

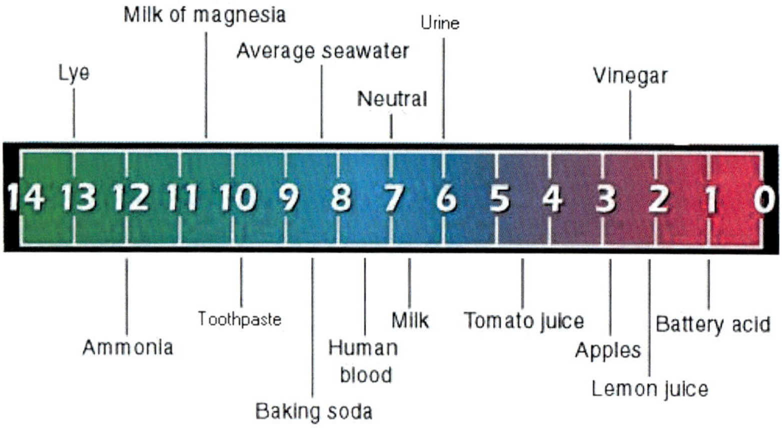

Learn more about your "Ultimate Personal Health Indicator" at

www.MagicOfpH.com

How's Your Diet? Test Your Urine pH!

HERE'S WHAT TO DO:

Pick any morning, first urination, when you've had at least 4-5 hours of sleep (or when you're first up for the day).

You'll need pH test strips, which are included in the pH Starter Packet available at www.WholeLifeWholeHealth.com.

1. Peel off a strip of yellow pH paper and run it through the urine stream, or dip it into a clean cup of urine.
2. IMMEDIATELY look at the wet paper and see what color matches the color guide most closely.
3. Make a note of the number on the color guide above the color you matched *(If the paper dries, the test isn't accurate, so check the pH strip right away).*

The goal for urine pH is to be on the alkaline side of the scale, but for the right reasons.

If the urine pH is below 6.0, you're done! You now know two things, 1) your diet is more acidic than alkaline, and 2) it's not an emergency. In time, symptoms will show up, little by little, that most people think are simply signs of growing older. Stiffness or sluggishness in the morning, short term memory lapses (have you ever walked into a room and forgotten why?), sagging, thinning or wrinkling skin are just some of the earliest signs of a body that is struggling with an acid overload. More vegetables and fruit plus whole food supplements like those already discussed will be needed to increase the pH level over time (this takes months).

If your pH is over 6.0, check it again the next morning. If the pH is still over 6.0, go to the next step.

For two days eat ONLY meats, dairy or grains. NO fruit or vegetables, including juices. If you are not a meat eater, concentrate on dairy and grains such as pasta, bread, and cereals.

Check the urine pH on the third morning as in steps 1-3 above. After two days of eating acid-forming foods, the urine should not even change the color of the pH paper! This means that you have adequate alkaline mineral reserves (mainly sodium and calcium) to neutralize (or "*buffer*") the acids in your diet. It also means that your normal diet is more on the alkaline side (that's why your reading was higher than 6.0 to start).

The recommendation for you is to keep eating lots of fruits and vegetables. When you stray occasionally, your body can handle it. *CONGRATULATIONS!*

Anything higher than 5.5 on the pH scale after two days of eating only acid-forming foods, means the alkaline mineral reserves are depleted and you're making ammonia to neutralize the acids in your diet.

The higher the number, the greater the urgency is to add vegetables and fruit to your diet, and slowly decrease the amount of meats, dairy and grains. In time, refined, processed or junk foods, and stimulants like caffeine or nicotine should be reduced or eliminated. This needs to be taken slowly if the numbers are higher than 7.0. Your level of toxicity is too high to make sudden, drastic changes. Start rejuvenating your liver *(see pages 11-32)* and monitor how you feel, in case protein needs to be added.

It's one thing to *believe* that you're doing a good job with your diet; it's another thing to *see* the truth! Use pH testing, **POSITIVE SIGNS TO LOOK FOR** (page 101), and the ***ALKALINE TRACKER***™ (page 110) to monitor the positive changes you make on your path to optimal health and wellness!

The **PH TEST PAPER,** which is included in the pH Starter Packet on www.WholeLifeWholeHealth.com, is essential to monitor pH. Follow the eating plan for rejuvenating your liver, found on pages 29-30 to alkalize your urine pH.

Most people *believe* they have healthy diets. Now you can test your belief!

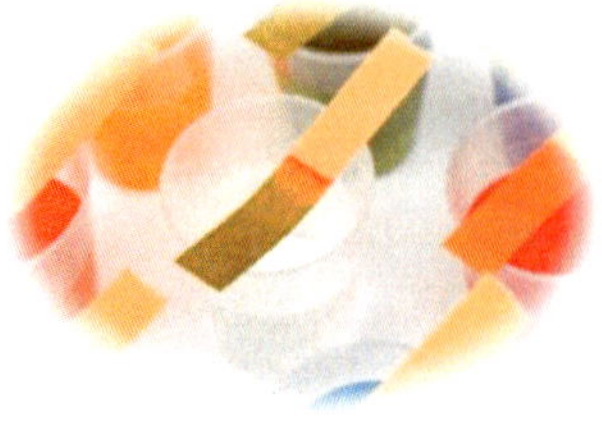

SALIVA pH: WORLD'S BEST "STRESS-O-METER"

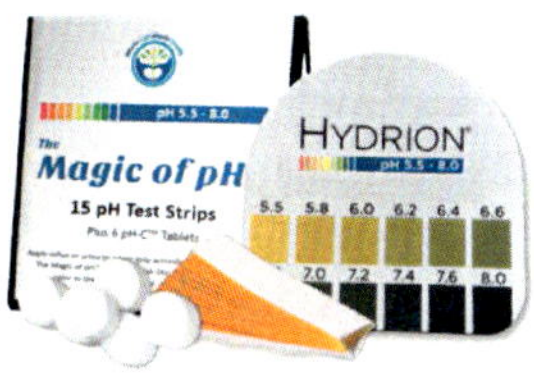

The environment in the mouth changes dramatically with foods and liquids, but since the 1970's, we've learned that saliva pH is one of the most accurate indicators of how stress affects the parts of the nervous system that control nearly every function of the body!

The "stress hormone," cortisol, made by the adrenal glands *(also known as the "stress glands")*, is most accurately measured in saliva fluid. Among other things, the adrenal glands produce adrenaline, a powerful hormone that is especially important for the "*fight or flight*" response, or "*emergency*" mode. Once an emergency – whether real or imagined – is over, the relaxed, "*healing*" mode should dominate. Both the body's *emergency* and *healing* systems may be evaluated by checking saliva pH.

As with urine pH, measuring saliva pH is simple, yet few people know how to perform the test properly, and even fewer know how to interpret the results. Learn more at www.MagicOfpH.com.

HOW TO TEST SALIVA pH

The goal for saliva pH is to be barely acidic (6.8) on the first part of the test, and alkaline (8.0) on the second part of the test.

You'll need pH-C TABLETS and pH TEST PAPER, both of which are found in the pH Starter Packet available at www.WholeLifeWholeHealth.com.

HERE'S WHAT TO DO:

Don't eat or drink anything except water for at least two hours before the test.

1. Tear off a strip of pH paper.
2. Place the paper on a tissue and hold the ends of the strip.

3. Next, form a puddle of saliva in your mouth and spit on the pH paper. This is not a delicate procedure; aim is everything!

Don't put the paper in your mouth, as the test won't be as accurate.

4. **IMMEDIATELY** look at the color of the paper, match it to a color on the pH scale, and note the corresponding number on the color guide.

This number reflects the current status of your emergency system. The lower the number, the more emergency activity is occurring.

The ideal result is 6.8.

5. Swish 1 teaspoon of freshly-squeezed lemon juice or a pH-C tablet in your mouth for a few seconds, until you taste the flavor throughout your mouth. The taste of the fresh lemon juice or pH-C tablet stimulates the production of saliva and should fill your mouth within a few seconds.

6. While you're swishing the pH-C tablet, tear off a second strip of pH paper and put it on a fresh tissue.

7. Spit out the pH-C tablet and swallow four times. Then, form another puddle of saliva in your mouth.

8. Hold the strip of pH paper on the tissue and spit on it, just like the first time. Immediately match the color of the paper with a corresponding number on the color guide.

This number reflects the current status of your *"healing"* mode. The higher the number, the more effectively your healing mode is functioning.

The ideal result is 8.0.

If you scored 6.8 or more on the first part of your saliva test, *CONGRATULATIONS!* You are handling the stresses of life relatively well.

If the second part of your saliva pH test was 8.0, *CONGRATULATIONS AGAIN!* Your healing mode is fully functioning.

Four Simple Steps
to Keep Your Body Alkaline

1. DRINK ALKALINE, IONIZED, "STRUCTURED" WATER

Since the 1970's, Alkaline Ionized, "structured" water, has been used in Japan to treat diseases in hospitals, promote overall health, and even eliminate germs that are resistant even to the strongest antibiotics! Today, individuals and families in the U.S. can make the same alkaline, ionized water at home!

Not only does Alkaline Ionized Water help alkalize the body, but ionization produces important antioxidant properties that other water does not have. Antioxidants have gained much attention in recent years, and have been the subject of volumes of research because of their cancer-fighting anti-aging effects.

The term, "structured," refers to the size of clusters into which water molecules arrange themselves. Due to their polarity, most water molecules are structured in clusters of 10-13 molecules, which is too big to penetrate our cells efficiently. Alkaline Ionized Water is broken into smaller clusters of five to six molecules, thereby enabling water to freely penetrate and hydrate every cell in the body.

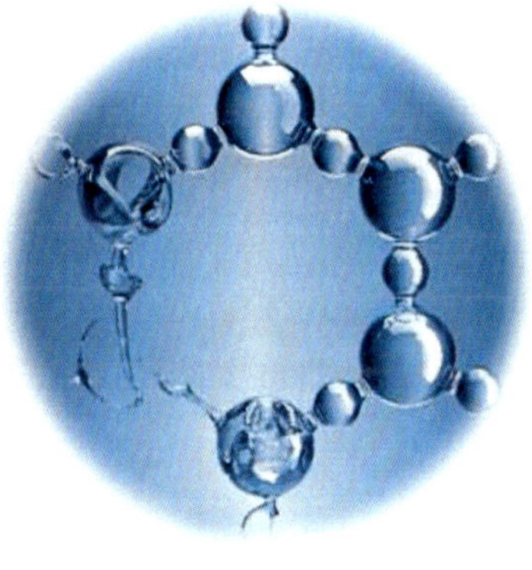

Alkaline, properly ionized and structured water was once abundant; however, as we began to pollute, treat, filter, or bottle our water, it lost the ionization and structure that imparts its life-enhancing and healing properties.

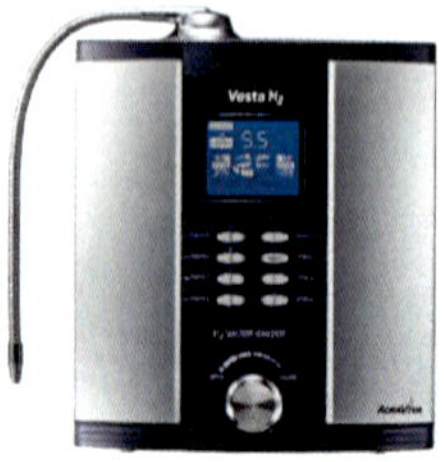

Restoring alkalinity, proper ionization and structure to your water at home is one of the easiest and most cost-effective ways to promote a healthier, more alkaline internal environment.

The mechanism for effectively creating alkaline water is by running ordinary water (first filtered of all impurities) through an electrolysis chamber that splits the water into two streams. One stream is alkaline and one is acidic. Alkaline water (pH of 8.5-9.5) is for drinking, and acid water (pH of 4.5-5.5) is for skin and hair care, cleaning and other uses. The unit we like best enables a range of pH choices for a variety of uses besides drinking, including cleaning produce, disinfecting, removing oils, watering plants, and replacing fabric softeners.

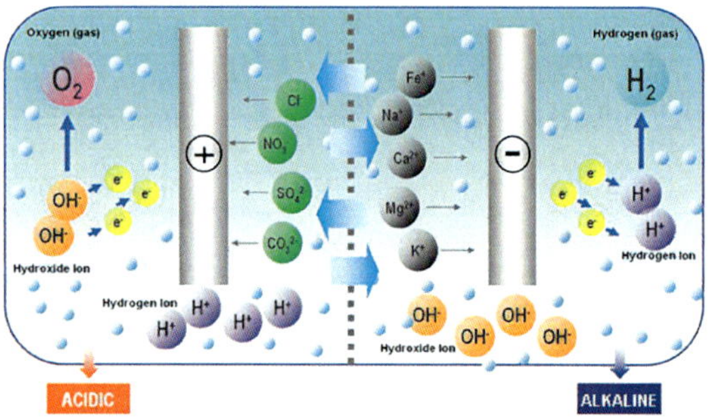

The systems we use and recommend to clients are made by a company that has perfected the technology, and calls the water produced by its systems, "H2" or "Hydrogen-Infused" water. Similar units available for home use in the U.S. are used in hospitals throughout Japan as approved medical devices, and are used to treat conditions and disinfect surfaces. More information may be found on our web site:

> **The initial investment is quickly recovered in savings over the cost of bottled water and other, less effective filters, to say nothing of the time, energy and money spent on therapies to correct the ravages of acid in the body!**

www.AlkalineWater.WholeLifeWholeHealth.com

2. EAT MAINLY ALKALIZING FOODS –

75% Vegetables and Fruit, 25% Nuts, Seeds, Grains, etc.

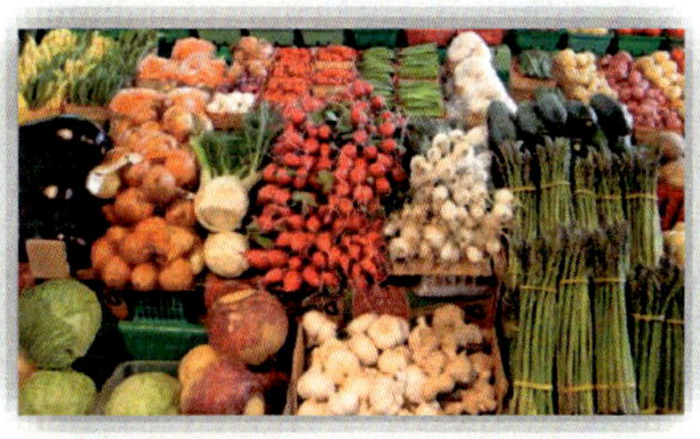

Dietary habits directly affect body chemistry. Every food or liquid has either an acidifying or alkalizing effect on the body after it has been digested.

In general, vegetables and fruits are alkalizing to the body (with a few exceptions), while nuts, seeds, grains, dairy, meats, poultry, fish, refined, processed and sugary foods have an acidifying effect (also with a few exceptions). A chart of acid-producing and alkalizing foods is available at YourPremiumWBC.wl-wh.com.

3. TAKE ALKALIZING, "WHOLE-FOOD" SUPPLEMENTS

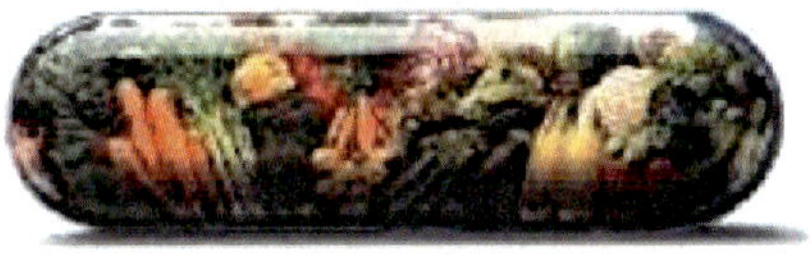

Foods by themselves simply cannot deliver the nutrition your body requires to thrive, and supplementation is critical to sustaining optimal health. Many vitamin formulas are actually stimulatory rather than health-enhancing. People may *feel* better for a while, but derive little real benefit!

We use and recommend only JUICE PLUS+® whole food concentrates. They provide nutrients as close to nature as possible; they have been shown to be recognized, absorbed, and utilized by the body for maximum benefit; and they provide a nutritional "*safety net*" to bridge the gap between what you *should* eat and what you *do* eat. Find them at www.WHOLELIFEWHOLEHEALTH.com.

> **CAUTION:**
> **Nutritional supplements are NOT created equal!**
> It doesn't matter what you take; it matters what your body *does* with what you

4. LEARN HOW TO "UPDATE" NEGATIVE EMOTIONS AND MEMORY

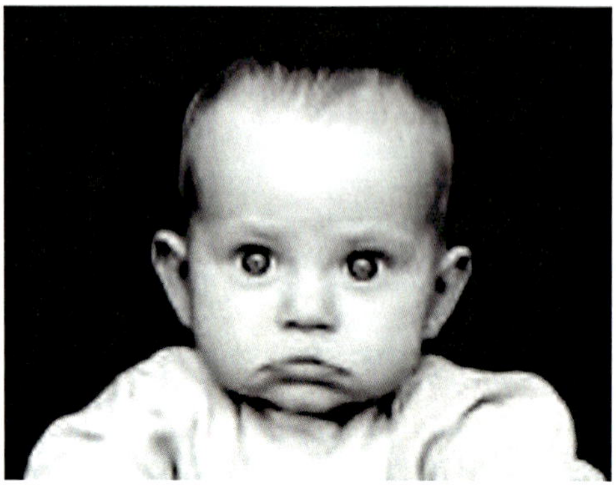

Emotional stress is most often overlooked as a major contributor to an acid body chemistry. Consider the following case history as a prime example of how powerful emotional stress can be:

A young aerobics instructor had a nearly perfect diet, supplemented with whole food concentrates, and her physical fitness regimen was ideal. She was the picture of health, but her bones were riddled with osteoporosis! She did everything "right," except that she was highly stressed emotionally, plagued by a constant feeling of anxiety. Once she began working with the techniques you're about to learn, her body stopped leeching minerals from her bones, and her bone density improved steadily over time.

Countless techniques have been developed over thousands of years in practically every culture to reduce, attempt to eliminate, or "manage" emotional stress. We recommend the **HEART, SOUL AND SPIRIT CLEANSE,** outlined in the next section. It is simple, effective and its steps can be performed anywhere and at anytime.

The Spirit-Mind-Body Connection

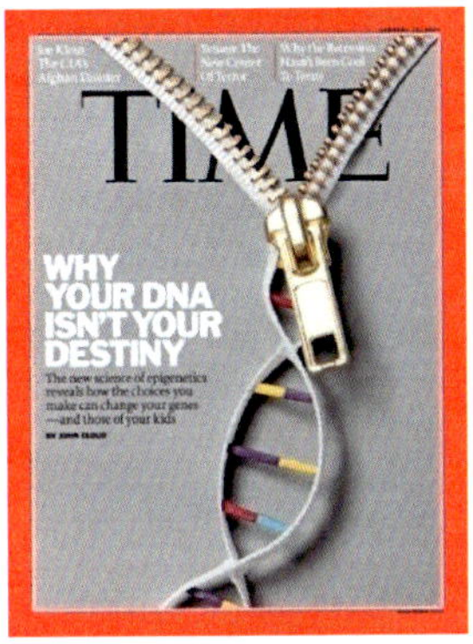

The relatively new science of epigenetics demonstrates what we observe throughout the wellness field: No matter who you are, where you're from, or the condition you're in, your state of health and well-being is more directly tied to your spiritual, mental, emotional, and nutritional environment than your family history or so-called genetic predisposition.

We often joke with clients, "If everyone in your family was a diabetic, you might not want to open an ice cream store, but it doesn't guarantee that you'll be a diabetic." Family history is only important when you repeat the habit patterns of your ancestors.

"For as he thinks within himself so he is."

(Proverbs 23:7, NASB)

The fact is that what you think, feel and believe is one of eight keys that can unlock your total health and well-being. Whether you acknowledge it or not, health and healing is intimately woven together with your thoughts, feelings and beliefs about yourself, your life, and, yes, even your relationship with God (or the absence of one).

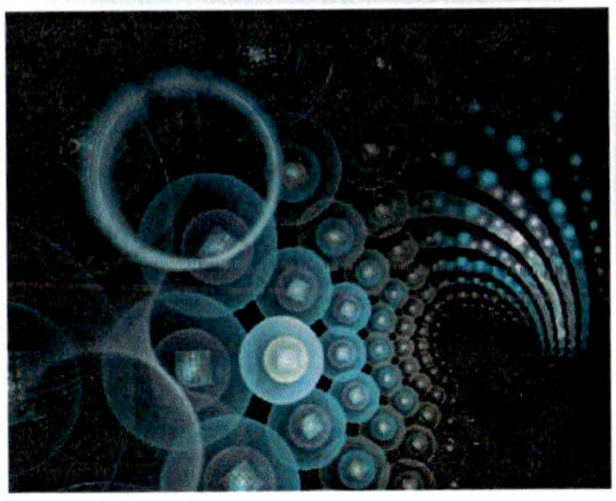

You develop "belief habits" as surely as you develop your nutritional habits. Quite literally, your framework for relating to God and how you view the purpose for your life, creates various patterns of thinking, feeling and believing. These patterns are shown to develop early in life, before you're capable of thinking for yourself; often they are self-limiting and are reinforced by your experiences. Everything about your life – especially your experience of its quality – is determined in large part by what you think about, what you *really* believe, and how you feel about both.

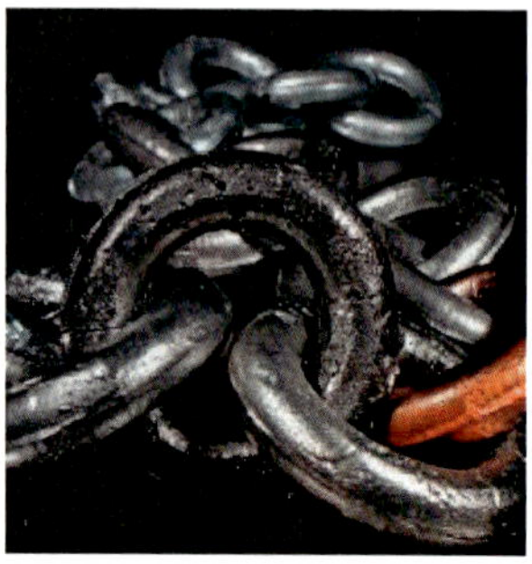

Since first being introduced to the so-called "*mind-body connection*" in a practical way in 1990, we have learned that it is much more profound; therefore, we refer to it as the "*spirit-mind-body connection.*" The "*Iron Rule*" of Cancer below, is one of the most startling applications of this concept.

Developed by the German physician, Ryke Geerd Hamer, after examining more than 15,000 cancer cases, the *Iron Rule* has never been disproved since Dr. Hamer first presented it in the late 1970s.

A SUMMARY OF THE "IRON RULE" OF CANCER

- **Every cancer starts with a brutal "psychic trauma" – a highly traumatic emotional shock – experienced by the person in a sense of profound loneliness, as the most serious event he or she has ever known.**
- **The way the person "colors" (interprets or feels about) the experience, determines the area of the brain that suffers a breakdown. Dr. Hamer was able to demonstrate this on MRI studies.**
- **The area of breakdown determines where tumor cells develop and proliferate.**
- **Even a cancer diagnosis can itself cause further trauma and additional areas of "breakdown."**
- **When the original insult or conflict was resolved, the "damaged" area in the brain began to wall itself off; the disease process was arrested, and healing began.**

*Note: The "Iron Rule" of Cancer is presented for information purposes only. We have seen the value of its principles in our own work with clients; however, we have no association with Dr. Hamer, or knowledge – much less endorsement – of any treatment methods he may use or teach.

Dr. Hamer's findings were corroborated independently by Dr. Brendan O'Reagan, in his study of "spon-taneous remission" in 10,000 cancer cases, published in 1993.

The connection between health and your thoughts, feelings, and beliefs, may seem far-fetched, compared with medical science. However, when obvious and consistent patterns appear while working with people of all ages and backgrounds, across a wide spectrum of conditions, and the results are so often dramatic, it is unthinkable to ignore or fail to share these vital principles.

Dr. Taylor realized, early on in practice, that his job was to help restore bodies, minds, and even spirits, to their original "blueprints." Time after time, he noticed that a kind of "short circuiting" in a person's sense of self worth and purpose was at the root of his or her pain, illness or dysfunction. Actual healing only began – and proceeded unhindered and unhampered – when thoughts, feelings and beliefs, which were incongruent or out of sync with a person's sense of inherent worth and divine design, were identified and corrected.

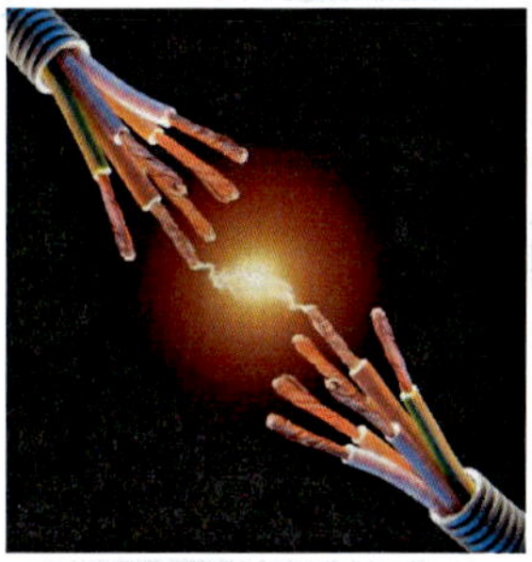

"Your faith has healed you." (Matthew 9:22, NIV)

It appears that the greater your faith, the greater your potential for, and the less you interfere with healing. Whatever *your* beliefs, be willing – only willing – to throw open the windows of your spirit, mind and heart to the possibilities of moving beyond your current horizons, and choose to live in the "*Realm of the Miraculous.*"

Heart, Soul and Spirit Cleanse

The order in which healing (or disease) seems to progress:

1. **SPIRIT** - through the emotions.
2. **SOUL** - through beliefs and memories contained in the mind.
3. **BODY** - the final expression – called symptoms – of what the spirit and mind contain.

The body is last in line and is only along for the ride.

One example to illustrate these principles:

A young woman, suffering from seizures several times a week for 18 months, had been forced to move back into her parents' home, quit her job, and stop driving. No medications had helped and she was understandably despondent.

In our first meeting, we identified an offending experience immediately prior to the onset of seizures. After a brief "re-timing" procedure, "short circuits" began to repair and seizures were replaced by a normally calm nervous system. Over the following hours, days, and weeks, the young woman's hope returned as her body restored its normal function. This true story illustrates a powerful principle:

Symptoms are the unpleasant and undesired responses to your thoughts, feelings and beliefs before, during and after experiences, which you wish were different, but which you were unable to change at the time.

The laws of healing — as well as pain and disease — seem to be universal. God designed within you an amazing process which, when recognized, honored, and followed, enables healing to occur, often beyond our ability to comprehend, let alone explain.

How it Works

How the trouble starts and what to do to move quickly from Emergency mode into Healing mode!

1. The inborn "*Emergency*" mode is triggered by an "*alarm bell,*" which sounds during an experience.

The emergency, *"fight-flight"* response, is automatic, utterly necessary for survival, and is evident even during development, as when a fetus responds violently to a sudden, loud noise. Outside the womb, alarms are triggered during events you wish weren't happening. Neurological, cardiovascular, hormonal, and other systems are stimulated in a cascade of responses, as emotions shift instantly from positive to negative.

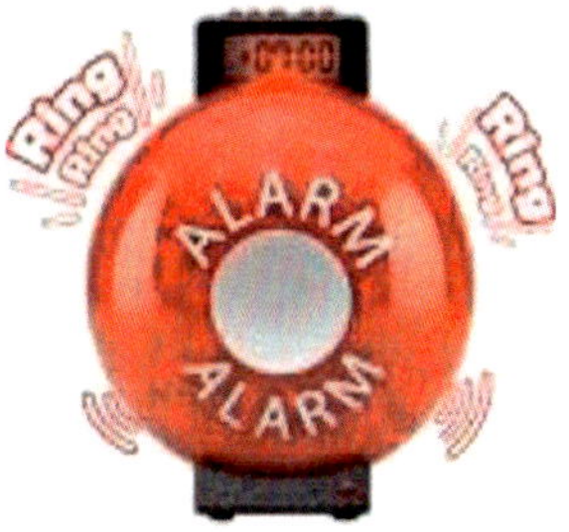

It's easy to ignore or dismiss the "alarm" consciously, treating the emotional shift as simply another in a long line of changes you don't like, but also don't address properly.

Ignored alarms, and the emotions associated with them, accumulate over time until they produce physical, mental or emotional changes that become symptoms you finally recognize as a problem. Initially, changes may be expressed subtly, such as in quality of sleep, food preferences or cravings, or even personality changes that others may notice and bring to your attention.

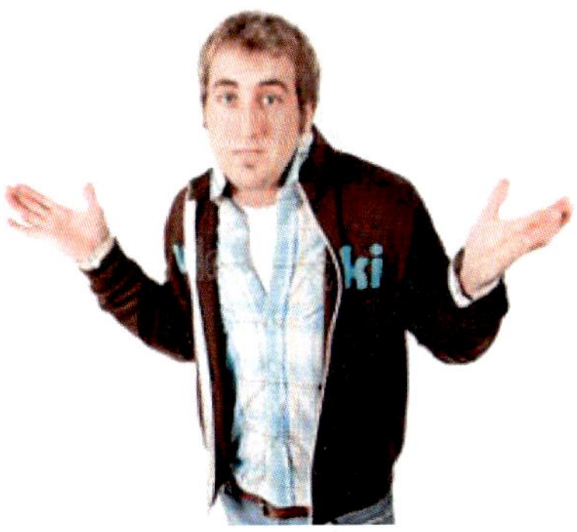

Pain, illness, or dysfunction is actually the body's *solution*; not the problem! Your job is to discover what problem is being solved!

Your body does not think, judge or reason; it's only along for the ride you provide. It will exhaust itself in an effort to survive both real and imagined emergencies: the alarm bells you don't turn off. Meanwhile, healing awaits your attention.

Drugs may help people feel better by changing symptom patterns, but the alarms that made them necessary continue unanswered. Ultimately, coping mechanisms that don't address the source of the alarms are no more effective than putting a pillow over an alarm clock or pulling the wire out of a warning light in your car.

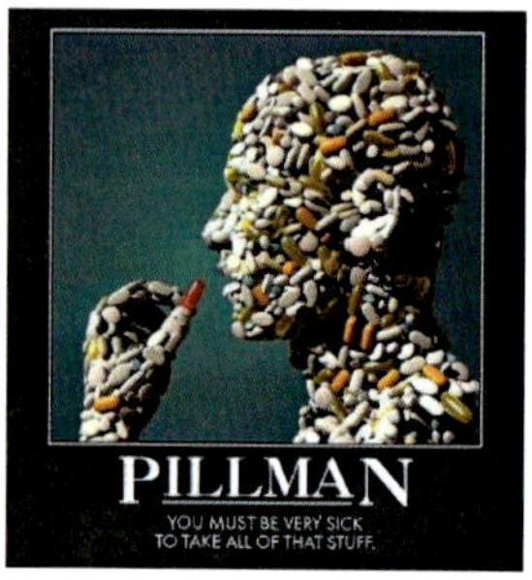

Survival and healing are mutually exclusive; they cannot operate simultaneously. Survival always takes precedence, until your lungs stop breathing and your heart stops beating. Death comes, by whatever means, when the survival response itself is exhausted.

2. **The experience that sounded the alarm is perceived sub-consciously as an "ambush." You didn't see it coming and, therefore, you couldn't have avoided it.**

Events that take you by surprise may be accompanied by thoughts such as, *"If only I had/hadn't...,"* or *"I should/shouldn't have..."* These thoughts come from limiting, blaming, and destructive, "flat earth" perspectives about yourself and your inherent worth. They support a belief that in some way you *deserve* the experiences you perceive as negative.

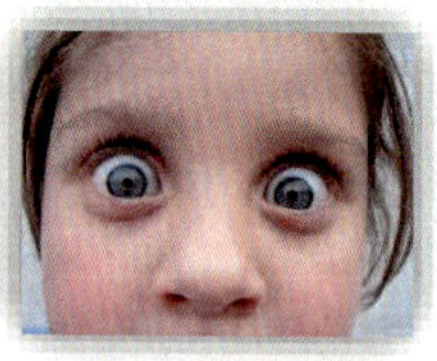

As you'll learn, unexpected things may happen and you may take "wrong turns," but they need not result in pain, illness, or dysfunction.

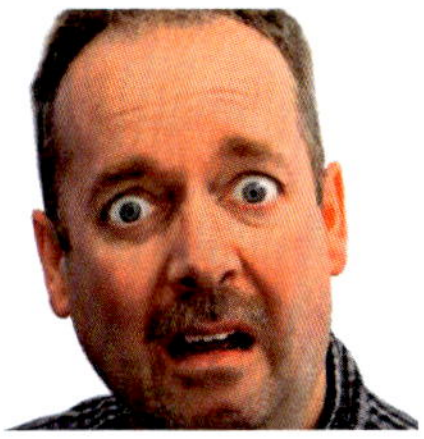

3. **Positive emotions *before* an ambush shift instantly to negative emotions *during* the experience. The sudden shift and the emotions are *completely normal*, but we cannot or do not express them at the time, so they turn inward.**

Ambushed positive feelings are far more important than negative emotions, when it comes to rapid healing. Once a positive emotion, such as joy, is "side-swiped," you may feel hurt, frustrated, or angry, but it usually doesn't stop there. You may turn bitter, disappointed over the past, and afraid of future experiences. You may begin "looking over your shoulders," and try to control your circumstances and others around you, in an attempt to guard against future ambushes. This is impossible, of course, and you waste valuable time and energy, while resisting many other rich human experiences and relationships.

As important as it is to resolve negative feelings, true healing lies in resolving the wounded positive emotions you were happily enjoying before the alarm sounded!

4. **Physical responses to the alarms – *symptoms* – are a survival response; a kind of "discharge" of ambushed positive feelings and unexpressed negative feelings.**

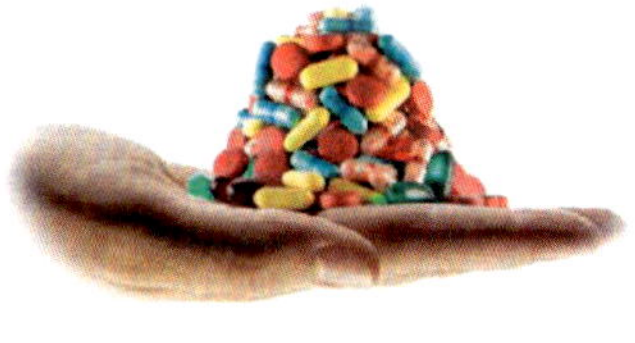

Any number of conditions may follow an unanswered alarm: colds, headache, fatigue, back pain, or something debilitating *(like seizures)* and even life-threatening *(like Dr. Hamer's cancer discovery)*. There are as many possibilities as there are parts of the body and compartments in the brain! In an effort to "control" or "cure" symptoms, many people fall into a seemingly endless pursuit of external treatments in a desperate search for true healing.

Symptoms are absolutely necessary to get our attention!

Six Steps to Rapid Healing

1. **Recognize that an "ambush" occurred. Even if you can't recall what the ambush was, recognition begins to quiet the "alarm" almost instantly.**

Experience has shown that healing cannot occur fully – and alarms will continue to sound – until you acknowledge three truths honestly in your heart:

> A. IT HAPPENED
> B. IT'S OVER
> C. IT'S OK NOW

A. IT HAPPENED. Something that was beyond your conscious control, turned on an alarm in the first place. *It is not critical that you recall consciously what "it" was.* Many experiences occur at such a young age that conscious recall may be impossible. Ambushes stored in memory can be released and their effects healed.

B. IT'S OVER. The message that whatever the emergency was is now over, must be perceived in the same area of memory as the original alarm, and with the same magnitude.

C. IT'S OK NOW. The coast is clear and it's safe again to, "*come out and play!*" Like a turtle poking its head out of the shell, you learn to trust again.

Faith makes trusting easier... It just does.

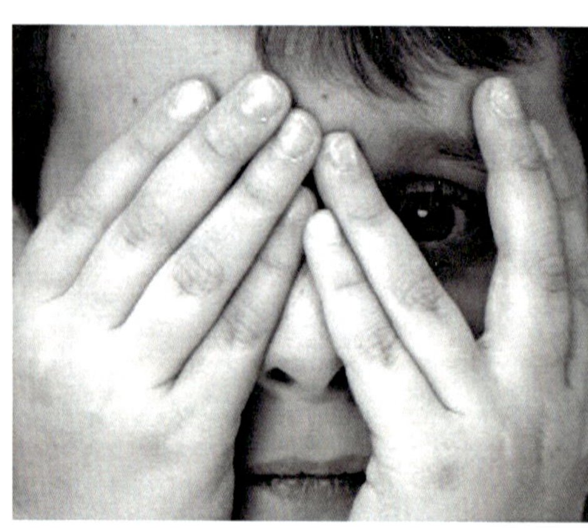

2. Evaluate your feelings after an "ambush" and your emotional state before the experience occurred.

Take it in two steps:

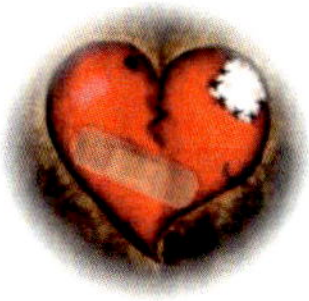

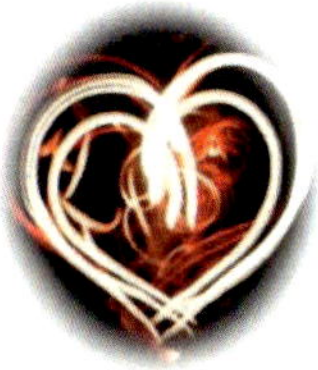

- Identify as many *negative* feelings as possible, *following* the ambush.
- Identify as many *positive* feelings as possible, *before* the ambush.

You do not have to *like* how an experience felt, and you don't have to volunteer for it again, but you must *acknowledge* it, and the feelings that accompanied it and preceded it. This calms the unresolved emotions and brings healing to the spirit.

If you *could* have responded any other way, you *would* have!

Your emotional responses at the time an experience occurs are normal and usually appropriate; however, they no longer need to continue after the ambush is over.

3. Change your mind, change your heart.

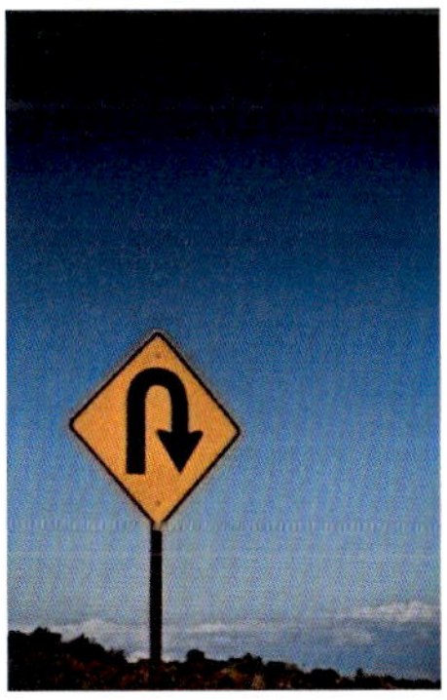

This step is *critical* to free you from suffering in a *"victim prison"* of your own making, and releases you into *willing* participation in the highest purpose for your life.

Changing your mind from thoughts that deny our inherent worth into those that affirm it – and changing your heart from feelings that chain you to bitterness, resentment, anger, blame, etc., into those of acceptance and forgiveness – enables you to live in peace, joy and delight!

Changing your mind – aka, "repentance" – requires that you recognize your accountability for what you do, think and say, and turn from *de*structive to *con*structive patterns. The sooner you take ownership of your part in any circumstance or relationship, the sooner you'll graduate to something better!

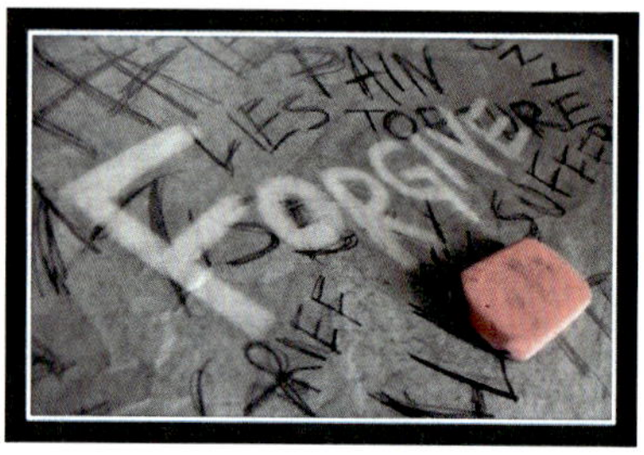

Changing your heart – aka "forgiveness" – works two ways: You must *give* it for what you perceive as the wrongs committed against you, and you must *receive* it for the wrongs you have committed.

Forgiving *does not* require you to like, agree with, or excuse anything that happened to you, or that you have done *(see the steps below)*.

FORGIVE = yield, concede, grant, relieve, exempt, free.

Forgiveness applies to others, yourself, and even to God. All three have been involved in the ambushes throughout your life. Forgiveness is simple, but not always easy; however, holding anything against anyone never affects them...it only makes *you* miserable!

HOW TO FORGIVE IN FOUR STEPS

Perform each step in the "theater of your mind," with feeling, for your own freedom's sake!

A. FORGIVE EVERYONE FOR EVERYTHING.

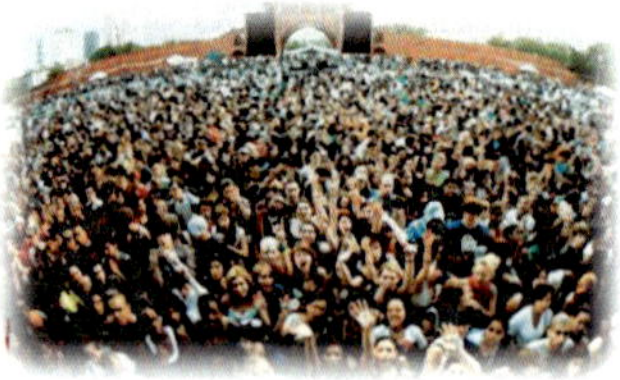

Line up everyone you've ever known across a huge stage and grant all pardon for everything. *Remember, this is for your sake, not theirs.* You'll be freeing yourself from all energy-wasting, forward progress-stopping resistance, resentment, and retaliation (even if it's silent and internal).

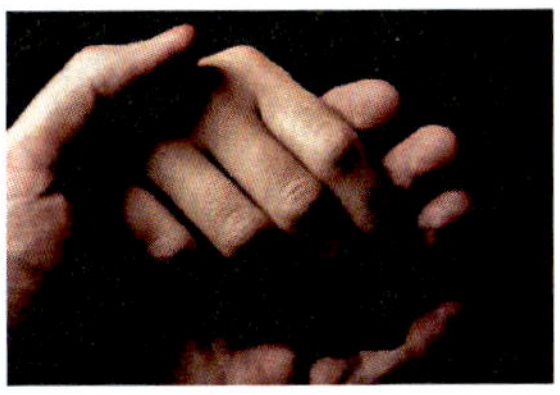

B. ASK EVERYONE TO FORGIVE *YOU*. Ask for amnesty and pardon for anything you *may* have done – a look, a word, or even just being in that place at that time. Even if you believe you were innocent in a situation, chances are that somewhere, sometime, you weren't, so give everyone permission to forgive you, and while you're at it, ask God to forgive you too.

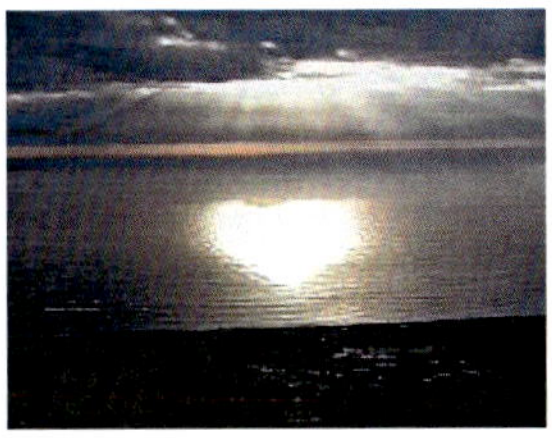

C. FORGIVE GOD. He can handle it, and holding against Him what you wish had not happened or wish had been different is the same as holding it against a person.

D. OWN YOUR "STUFF," REPENT, AND FORGIVE YOURSELF for carrying around the effects of the ambushes and the unanswered alarms in your body, soul, and spirit. Recognize, accept, and acknowledge where you missed the mark; then turn and choose a more excellent way.

A COUPLE QUICK NOTES:

- You may never actually speak to anyone. This process is accomplished within yourself, because that's where the alarm sounded in the first place.

- This is serious business, the result of which is nothing short of your total freedom and release – spiritually, mentally, and physically – from a prison you built; a prison of resentment, bitterness, guilt, shame, disappointment, despair, blame, and more, from all of which you may now walk away...*FREE!*

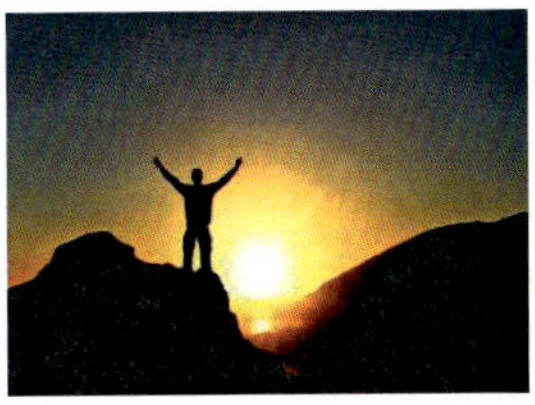

"Forgive, and you will be forgiven."
(Luke 6:37, NIV)

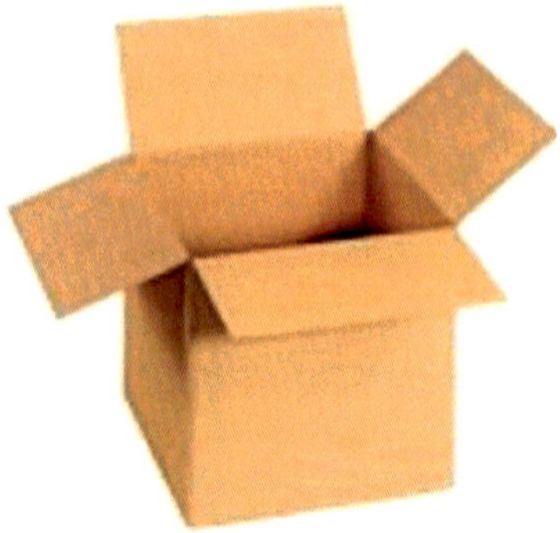

4. **Release the past. Fill a box with the experiences you wish hadn't happened or wish had been different, and set it at God's feet!**

Putting your experiences in a big box and leaving it at God's feet releases the burden of your past to the One Who can handle it!

Throw anything in the box that no longer serves you, from the earliest childhood hurts to the most recent challenges. Whatever you no longer want to carry or drag behind you goes in the box.

Once the box is loaded, all that is left is to close the flaps, tape it up, or tie a bow around it, and step back.

> ***"Come to Me, all who are weary and heavy-laden, and I will give you rest."*** (Matthew 11:28, NASB)

To go free, simply look God "in the eye," and say, "*Thank You,*" for what you learned from your experiences and what you're learning now *(even if you don't know what it is!)*. Reciting this statement may be all you are capable of at first, but, if you apply the preceding steps well, one day you'll truly feel thankful.

When you fully recognize and appreciate the priceless jewels in your life today – the relationships and experiences that you wouldn't trade for anything – you can truly say, "*Thank You*" to God for what His love and purpose required, and feel genuinely glad for the price that was paid.

> **When you are more grateful than you were ever hurt, you're free. Healing then becomes inevitable and unstoppable!**

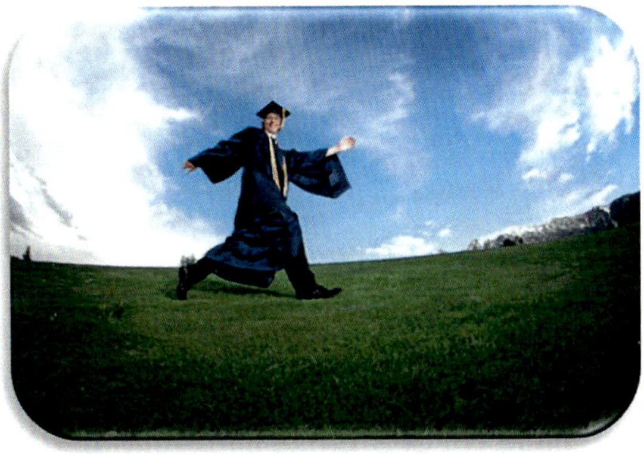

5. Receive your diploma...with honors!

The first four steps of this process – recognition, repentance, forgiveness, and release with gratitude – transform experiences of pain, dishonor, or shame, into victories that qualify you for "graduation" with honors.

You're free! You're on the "other side," living free, and living the victory! This applies not only to physical healing, but to healing in every area of your life.

Now it's up to you to live, minute-by-minute and hour-by-hour, in ways which agree with, support, and reinforce your new "status," *no matter what anyone else says or does,* until it becomes integrated into the fabric of your character.

You have moved from victim to victor and now it's time to, ***"put on the new [humanity], created to be like God in true righteousness and holiness"*** (Ephesians 4:24, NIV).

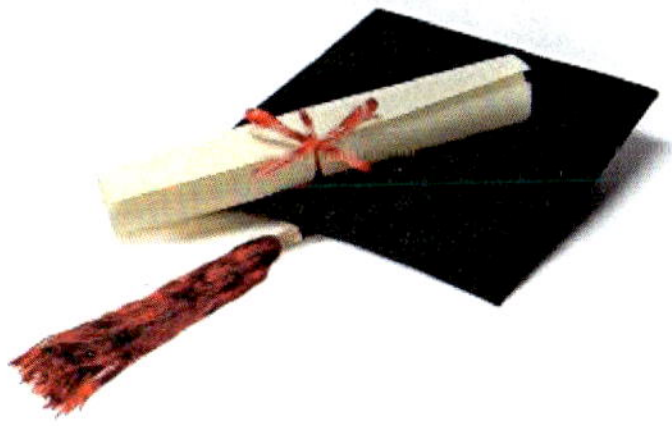

What does *that* look like?
How does *that* feel?

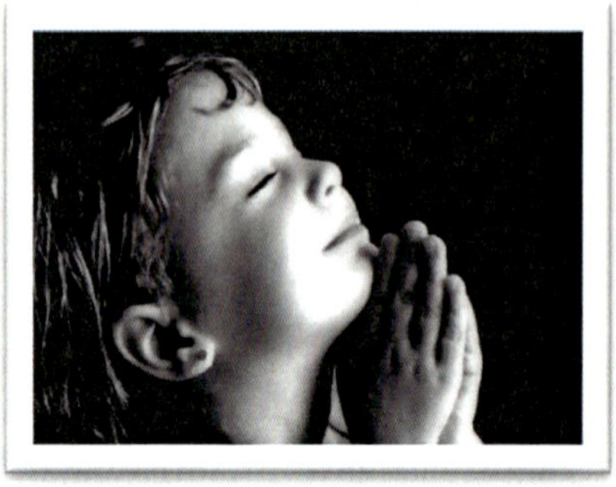

6. Establish the continual, conscious exercise of your spirit.

Sometimes, your life might feel like you're a passenger with no one at the wheel of your own vehicle. You have a "death grip" on the dashboard, as if your life is careening out of control.

You have an opportunity today to move into the driver's seat, with a *"life grip"* on the steering wheel, negotiating turns, high-ways and alleys, with greater ease as your skills improve.

The most valuable instruments to guide you – like a spiritual *"GPS"* – are the Scriptures. Unique among the world's volumes of religious writing, the Old and New Testaments are, *"God revealing Himself to mankind,"* as Adlai Loudy described in his 1926 book, *God's Eonian Purpose*; as opposed to other writings, which are, *"man's attempt to explain his god."*

Believe what you like, the principles contained in the Scriptures provide reliable road maps for total daily health habits, including spiritual ones. If this seems a bold, if not incredible statement, it is based on decades of combined experience in helping people restore and sustain their health and well-being, contrary to most of the conventional wisdom.

Learning to be directed by the Holy Spirit has proven 100 percent successful in providing a foundation for levels of peace and ease that translate into profound physical and mental health and well-being.

> ***"I will send him to you...the spirit of truth will be guiding you into all the truth."*** (John 16:8, 13)

The more you remind yourself of who you are to God, according to His own word, the more grateful you become for everything that has been or is today a part of your life. The more you guard this awareness, the more alert you will be when "alarm bells" sound; you will hear them sooner and act on them quicker. You become more loving, accepting, and forgiving of yourself and others. You discover how that improves your physical, mental, and emotional health, and also your relationships at home, at work, and at play. In time, you may even learn possibly the best lesson in preventive health care: ***"Do not judge so that you will not be judged"*** (Matthew 7:1, NASB).

> ***"Beloved, I pray that in all respects you may prosper and be in good health, just as your soul prospers."*** (3 John 2, NASB)

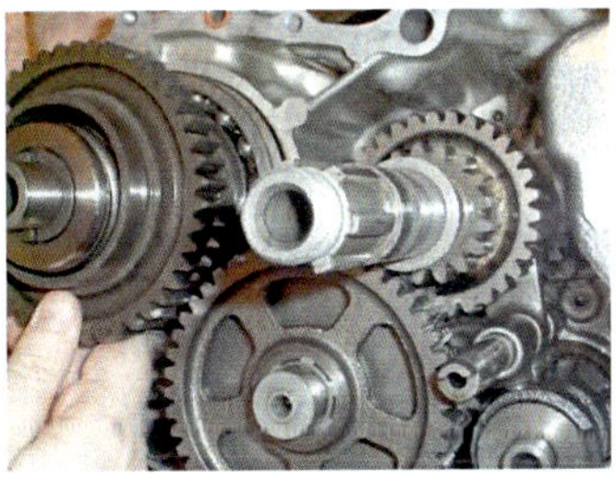

ALL TOGETHER NOW

HOW IT WORKS (from pages 71-81):

1. An "*alarm bell*" sounds in your spirit during an experience.
2. The experience is perceived subconsciously as an "ambush."
3. Positive emotions *before* an ambush turn to negative emotions *during* the experience, and stay that way until you resolve them.

4. Physical symptoms are a *survival response* — a kind of "discharge" of ambushed positive feelings and unexpressed negative feelings.

SIX STEPS TO RAPID HEALING (from pages 74-81):

1. **"IT HAPPENED!"** – Recognize that an "ambush" occurred, even if you can't recall what it was.
2. Identify as many *positive* emotions *before* the "ambush" as possible, and as many *negative* emotions as possible *when* it occurred.
3. **"IT'S OVER!"** – Repent and forgive. Changing your mind from past thoughts, beliefs and actions is critical! Then, ask for and receive forgiveness, and freely forgive others, including God.
4. **"IT'S OK NOW!"** – Fill a box with the experiences you wish hadn't happened or wish had been different, and place it at God's feet. Say, *"Thank You for what I learned,"* until you *feel* it. When you succeed in this step, you're free!
5. Receive your "graduation diploma." Well done!
6. Establish the continual, conscious exercise of your spirit; the single most important step to sustain optimal overall health and well-being.

REVIEW AND REPEAT FREQUENTLY

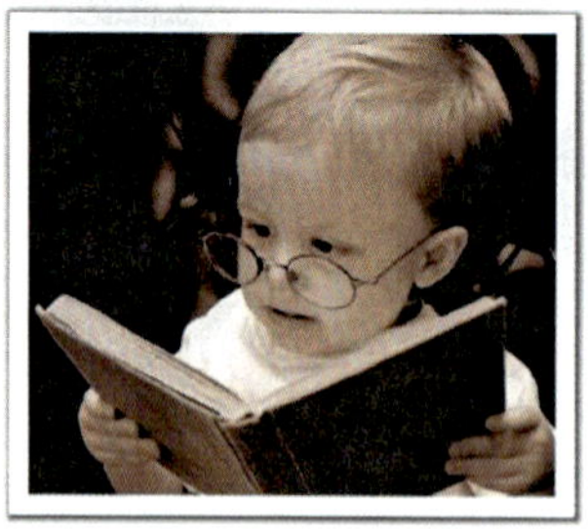

Experiences you wish were different are likely to happen, and memories of past events and relationships may surface. You can achieve healthier responses to future "ambushes" by using "**HOW IT WORKS**" to maintain a healthy perspective, and **SIX STEPS TO RAPID HEALING** to release any ill effects and promote maximum spiritual, mental, and physical well-being.

Miracles Await Your Recognition and Reception

Permanent healing seems to depend on your willingness to recognize and receive the miracles happening in and around your life all the time. Sometimes, the miracles you want aren't the ones you most need to recognize and receive first. The simple fact is, however, the more you look, the more you'll find; the more you find, the more there are to discover. It's a skill you can develop.

Recognizing and receiving miracles results in unshakable confidence in your true worth, and a constant state of appreciation, wonder, reverence, and even worship

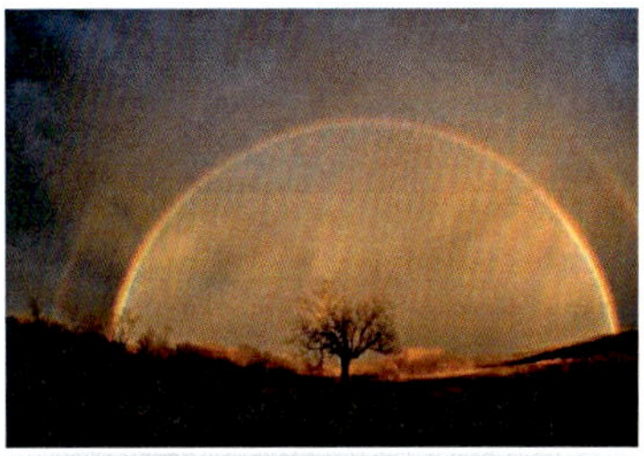

Who Restores Sight to the Blind?

Barbara was once the Keynote Speaker for a world convention at the newly completed National Soccer Stadium in Abuja, Nigeria. Many in the audience had walked for miles to hear the word of God. After Barbara finished speaking, people were invited to come forward for prayer. An 18-year-old boy, who was blind from birth and known to many who had come hoping for his miracle, was pushed to the front of the line.

The boy's eyeballs were pure white...no cornea, iris, or pupil.

As Barbara laid her hands on the boy, praying for him in the name of Jesus, *the boy's eyes began to form and he began to see!*

Barbara asked the boy, *"What do you see?"*

He replied, *"I see shapes! I see fingers! I see you!"*

"How do you feel?" Barbara asked.

"I feel happy."

The stadium erupted in spontaneous praise to God for the miracle everyone had witnessed.

That young boy had probably prayed for sight countless times before that night. Many others had probably prayed for him and laid hands on him too. Barbara's faith in God, coupled with the boy's, met the Lord's power and purpose that night.

Miracles can't be bought. God created something out of nothing, in front of tens of thousands of witnesses – and thousands more would hear or read the story later (as you are now) – for God's glory.

Read this story again and let the significance sink into a mind that may not comprehend...

...how a boy born blind received working eyeballs and the gift of sight to go with them!

Who can form working eyes? Jesus of Nazareth can! (Read the story of Jesus and the blind man in John 9.)

The truth is, you too can live in the *Realm of the Miraculous*!

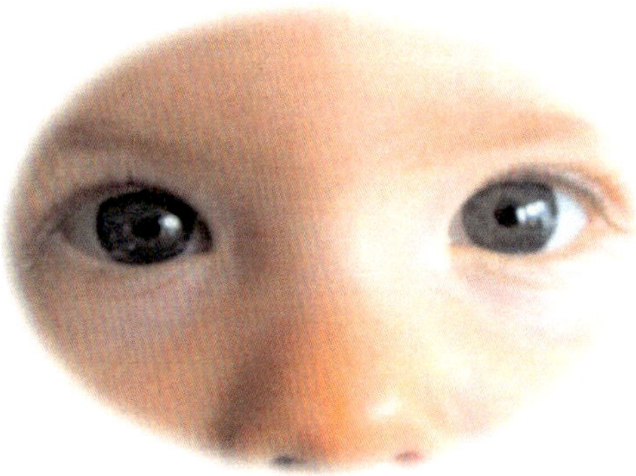

"With men it is impossible, but not with God, for all is possible with God."
(Mark 10:27)

Dr. Taylor Traces the Steps of a Miracle

A desperate mother called to say that her daughter was lying in a well-known hospital, and three days of intravenous drug therapy had failed to stop a deadly meningitis bacterial infection. After a week of "doctor-hopping," the hospital's Chief of Infectious Disease was overseeing the case.

"Is there anything you can do?" the mother asked.

"What was her first symptom?" I asked.

A symptom is often the first evidence of an ongoing alarm.

"She came home with a sore throat on Tuesday, but she was fine before that." Mom continued, *"The doctors looked for Strep, Lyme, Lupus, Mononucleosis, Guillain-Barre; you name it, but her condition only worsened. She developed head pain, fever, and even began hemorrhaging under the skin around her joints."*

The hospital doctors were now concerned for the daughter's life, since intravenous antibiotics had no effect after three days *(the drugs were safe to administer for a maximum of seven days).*

As I listened to the story, I "saw" by the spirit what had happened and that the process could be reversed.

We found the source of the alarm – the "ambush" – using the body's first symptom as a signal.

I said, *"Your daughter had an enormously stressful experience, during which she either wanted to scream or say something, and couldn't. That's what started the sore throat."*

The body's survival response escalated as the unresolved emotions continued to trigger the alarm.

"Your daughter perceived the experience as life-threatening; it overwhelmed her immune system, allowing the bacteria to grow. You have the same bacteria in your spinal fluid, but your immune system keeps it in check.

"What must happen now is that the message, 'the emergency is

over,' has to be received in the same area of the brain where the alarm was first sounded, and with the same intensity. Healing will begin immediately as your daughter's immune system stops responding to the emergency, and resumes its normal function."

The alarm stopped as quickly as it began.

Later that evening, in her hospital room, the daughter thought of the feeling(s) she had at the time the "emergency" occurred. We took her through steps of forgiving those involved for everything they did to contribute to the emotions that had overwhelmed her. She forgave herself for her response that compromised her well-being; and she received forgiveness from everyone involved for any part she played in the situation. Finally, she forgave God for what His purpose and love for her required. All this was done silently and internally on the daughter's part.

Finally, she placed the whole experience at God's feet, wrapped and sealed in a box. In her mind's eye, she looked at Him and said, *"Thank You. Thank You for what I learned from this experience. Thank You that the emergency is over. I am now safe in Your love and care."*

Healing began immediately.

Within a few minutes, a very sick young lady was able to lift and turn her head without pain. By the next day, she was up and walking, and left the hospital two days later with a clean bill of health.

She recognized and received the miracle, even though it was denied by others.

The medical staff was ecstatic that the "miracle of modern medicine" had finally worked, but the family knew that God had performed the real miracle.

To God be the glory!

I was not at the daughter's bedside during the steps outlined above. I met her for the first time five days later. The **HEART, SOUL AND SPIRIT CLEANSE** was accomplished over the telephone!

Five Reasons
Why Healing May Be Elusive or Short-lived

1. You have more invested in your condition than in healing.
2. You have more invested in pleasing others than in being healthy.
3. There is a higher "TOP PRIORITY" for healing.
4. An ongoing stimulus interferes with healing.
5. "Infirmity" serves a higher purpose.

1. You have more invested in your condition than in healing.

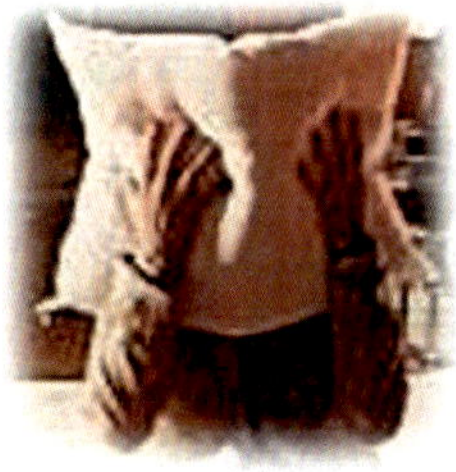

Some people will actually reject healing in favor of pain, illness, or dysfunction, because they fear losing the attention they are receiving from being sick more than they value healing. We've worked with clients who were within reach of a real breakthrough, and who chose to reject it.

- **A woman rushed up to the stage after a workshop, and *proudly* listed her diseases and medications, like they were pictures of her kids! The principles we shared had fallen on deaf ears.**
- **A client whose debilitating headaches of 40 years disappeared in six weeks, stopped coming because, he said, *"I just can't believe they can be gone that easily."* His headaches returned, fulfilling his belief.**
- **Another client, who had improved rapidly, announced that she could not continue. She said, *"If I get any better, my husband will stop doing everything for me."***

The healing power within you works when you accept it and adopt a spirit of gratitude for its perfection. When the personal "payoff" of infirmity – better known as self-pity – is greater than the perceived benefit of healing, some may reject the possibility of experiencing a miracle and deny themselves the opportunity to heal.

2. You have more invested in pleasing others than in being healthy.

Well-meaning family and friends may give advice freely, believing that they are "*just trying to help,*" but the result can sometimes be tragic. Here's just one example:

A colleague and friend, with as healthy a lifestyle as anyone we knew, once asked for help with what had become a life-threatening illness. She had pursued conventional treatment at the insistence of her family, and by the time we began working together, she had been under medical care for months, with a poor prognosis for recovery.

We quickly identified the cause of the "alarm" and, using the **HEART, SOUL AND SPIRIT CLEANSE,** she began to improve immediately. Her appetite returned, and she gained strength and stamina over a few short weeks, while continuing conventional drug therapy. She even began planning to return to work.

Then something happened: Following a visit from some of her family, our friend's condition deteriorated rapidly. It was as if her celebration of renewed strength and vitality had been swept from underneath her feet.

The conflict inside her was obvious when we saw our friend for what proved to be the last time. Without speaking a word, we knew she had resigned herself to follow her family's wishes. The miracle that had been operating powerfully stopped abruptly. She died a few weeks later.

Even if no one in your life welcomes the healing miracle you experience, guard it!

> **"...that which is committed to you, guard..."** (1 Timothy 6:20)

Pleasing others may cost you more than you would ever want to pay. If you care more about making others feel better than you do about being well, you run the risk of turning your back on a miracle. When you face a choice between trusting God and trusting man, trust God.

3. There is a higher, "TOP PRIORITY" for healing.

Bodies heal according to internal priorities that may not match your conscious "checklists." Healing doesn't always begin where you feel the need, but in the area of the greatest immediate threat to your survival. Here's an example:

A 90-year-old man with painful hands and wrists, believed he had carpal tunnel syndrome. After working with him for two weeks, he reported no change; *"But,"* he said, *"I can sure go up and down stairs without knee pain now."* He had never reported a knee problem and we had no idea that his knees were hurting!

The principle of **TOP PRIORITY** became apparent, as the innate, inborn intelligence in the man's body worked to heal his knees first, because they were more important to his survival at the time than his hands and wrists.

Just remember:
"Trust the process."

Skeptics sometimes voice a paradigm known as, *"the limitations of matter,"* the premise of which is that healing is subject to certain physical limitations.

Under this belief, the boy in Nigeria would never have received his sight; the 70-year-old man whose neck appeared fused with arthritis on X-rays, would never have regained his flexibility; the woman with rods implanted alongside her spinal column would never have enjoyed hiking mountains again; the woman whose rotator cuff muscles had been torn, literally, from their attachments, would never have trimmed her hedges that summer.

Healing is a process, not a destination, but it is inevitable when interference with its normal expression has been removed.

Beliefs have more to do with your well-being than you often realize. Experiences like those above have convinced us never to place limits on your body's God-given healing potential.

4. An ongoing stimulus interferes with healing.

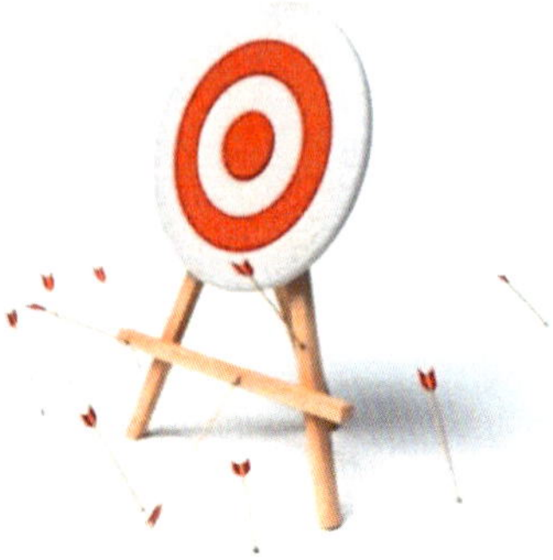

The doctor who first inspired Dr. Taylor once said, *"If you leave my office and go out to eat a hamburger or get mad at someone on the way home, you'll undo the good we just did."* In other words, when healing stops or never seems to begin, and the three previous possibilities have been eliminated, rather than conclude that you're defective or unlucky in some way, consider looking at what you're doing to interfere with the process. This principle is similar to **TOP PRIORITY**, except that your choices in some area(s) of life are creating a greater survival priority than healing.

The most common question we hear when we finish our first meeting with someone who has tasted the possibilities of a victorious life is, *"How long will this last?"* Our answer is always the same:

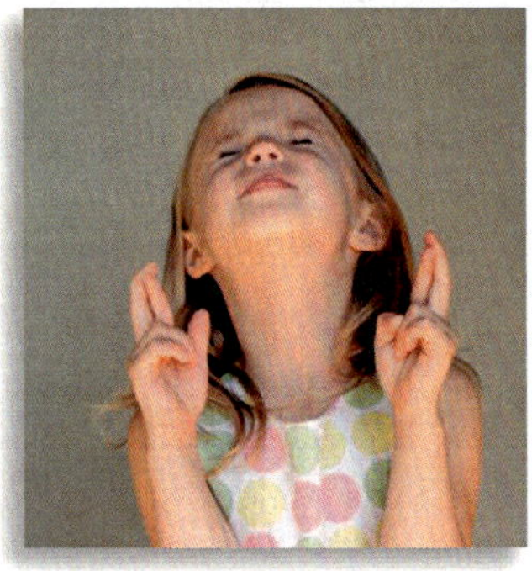

"Your body will respond perfectly to the choices you make. If you do everything you've always done, you'll get what you've always had. If, however, you make a spiritual commitment to yourself; if you take ownership of the only body and the only life God has given you, and be committed to serving the highest purpose for your life in every area, you can walk in divine health. It's up to you."

Your choices ultimately determine the course and speed of healing, so if healing isn't happening, examine your choices.

5. Infirmity serves a higher purpose.

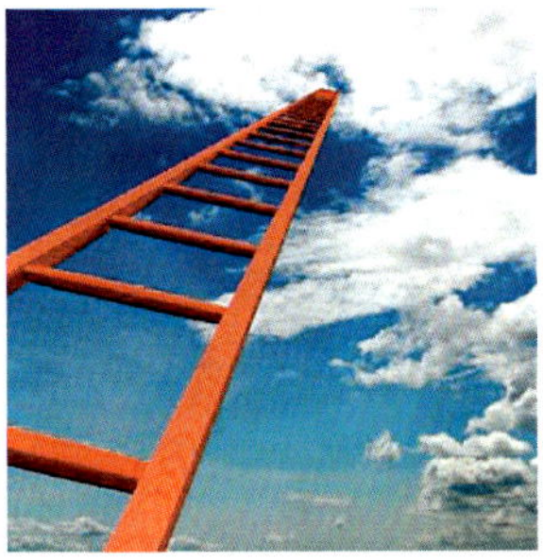

Why do some people heal and some don't, when all of the previous possibilities have been addressed? The phenomenon of an infirmity serving a higher purpose may be rare, and requires a leap of faith to accept; however, it is not unprecedented.

A man was troubled for many years by a condition for which he sought but never found relief. He figuratively called the problem a "splinter in the flesh," and as a man of great faith, he prayed three times to have the "splinter" removed. The Lord told the man that His grace was enough, so he wore it as a badge of honor; people would have to look past his appearance to hear the message that Paul of Tarsus brought *(read 2 Corinthians 12)*.

Another man was merely plain-looking, but people rejected and despised him. He was said to be a man of suffering, familiar with pain, and seemingly afflicted by God; but his message was compelling, convicting, and promising, all at the same time. He was eventually killed for what he knew and shared with others. His life and teachings are still studied and even followed by billions of people worldwide. His name was Jesus of Nazareth *(read Isaiah 53)*.

Barbara's body was once ravaged by muscular dystrophy and she was flat on her back one day, when she prayed for God's purpose – rather than her own – to be fulfilled in her life. Until then, she had no motivation to pray like that, much less hear the Lord's voice weeks later, when He told her to start walking. God permanently healed Barbara for His purpose and she is a walking miracle today. Her story has inspired audiences all over the world, lifting them to see beyond their current horizons. Read about it and watch the video on her website, *www.BarbaraBrown.com*.

How to Identify Top Priorities

Whether it's getting rid of headaches or improving relationships, this simple form can help stimulate and focus your thinking, activate your memory, and help you determine clearly the top priorities for what you most want to work better in your life.

Once the priorities are identified, apply the steps on pages 81-82 to identify and remove any interference between you and the innate healing potential that God created in you.

Dating these forms is a great way to track success!

DATE: ____________________________

Top 3 Health Challenges (physical, mental, emotional or spiritual):
Example: Seizures

______________________ ______________________ ______________________

When did each of these begin?
Example: 18 months ago

______________________ ______________________ ______________________

What major event happened in your life at that time?
Example: Dental visit – Dr. and assistant were pre-occupied during procedure

______________________ ______________________ ______________________

What negative feeling(s) do you associate with that event?
Example: Neglected, angry, frustrated, impatient

______________________ ______________________ ______________________

What positive feeling(s) do you recognize prior to that event?
Example: Happy, expectant, hopeful, relaxed

______________________ ______________________ ______________________

SAMPLE EMOTIONS TO "STIR THE POT"

NEGATIVE EMOTIONS

1. Embarrassed
2. Abused
3. Ridicule
4. Shame
5. Guilt
6. Bitterness
7. Regret
8. Remorse
9. Anger
10. Hate
11. Pride
12. Judgment
13. Indecisive
14. Selfish
15. Depressed
16. Demanding
17. Immoral
18. Critical
19. Resentment
20. Vulnerable
21. Abandoned
22. Suspicious
23. Worry
24. Fear
25. Dishonest
26. Doubt
27. Bored
28. Upset
29. Repulsive
30. Paranoia
31. Unfaithful
32. Indignant
33. Impatient
34. Rejected
35. Rejecting
36. Irritated
37. Cynical
38. Greed
39. Obsessed
40. Powerless
41. Anxious
42. Spiteful
43. Lonely
44. Concerned
45. Dominated
46. Jealous
47. Grudge
48. Argumentative
49. Compulsive
50. Fighting
51. Ruthless
52. Submissive
53. Inadequate
54. Devastated
55. Indifferent
56. Dread
57. Despair
58. Resignation
59. Frustrated
60. Persecuted
61. Envy
62. Destructive
63. Unloved
64. Self-Pity
65. Grief
66. Striving
67. Lethargic
68. Disgraced
69. Worthless
70. Humiliated
71. Apathy
72. Hostile
73. Tolerate
74. Blame
75. Defilement
76. Degradation
77. Loss
78. Poverty
79. Manipulated
80. Demeaned
81. Humiliation
82. Controlled
83. Betrayed
84. Denial

POSITIVE EMOTIONS

1. Love
2. Joy
3. Peace
4. Patient
5. Kind
6. Faithful
7. Goodness
8. Gentle
9. Self-Control
10. Passion
11. Stable
12. Trust
13. Careful
14. Harmonious
15. Warm
16. Glad
17. Intimacy
18. Friendship
19. Perfection
20. Elated
21. Grateful
22. Tranquility
23. Delight
24. Creative
25. Accepting/Accepted
26. Inspired
27. Hopeful
28. Unwavering
29. Conscientious
30. Devoted
31. Satisfied
32. Gratified
33. Honest
34. Happy
35. Calm
36. Adoring
37. Amiable
38. Agreeable
39. Compatible
40. Expectant
41. Right
42. Composure
43. Dedicated
44. Serenity
45. Quiet
46. Consistent
47. Content
48. Enjoyment
49. Fulfilled
50. Cherish
51. Desire
52. Sensitive
53. Imaginative
54. Enthusiastic
55. Gracious
56. Blissful
57. Loyal
58. Comfort
59. Reliable
60. Truthful
61. Eager
62. Excited
63. Respect
64. Compassion
65. Pleased
66. Encouraged
67. Understood
68. Dependable
69. Exacting
70. Curious
71. Empathy
72. Recognized
73. Exhilaration
74. Holy
75. Innocent
76. Clarity
77. Security
78. Abundance
79. Restored
80. Purity
81. Celebrated
82. Flow
83. Believe
84. Faith

Charts adapted in part from the book, *Feelings Buried Alive Never Die*, by Karol K. Truman

Five Simple Rules For the New You

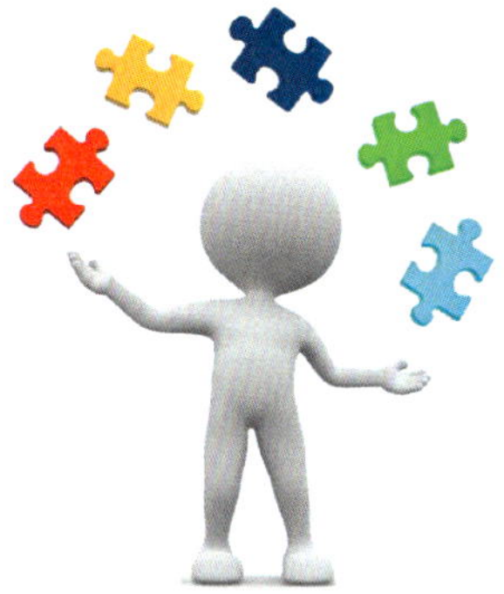

- **SHOW UP.** Some authorities say 90 percent of success is showing up...daily, hourly, to who you are and the purpose for which you were created, wherever you are, whatever you do, and whomever you're with. One motivational speaker says it this way: *"Be where you are, boy!"*

- **PAY ATTENTION.** Listen for and obey the quiet but distinct voice in your spirit, leading you to take steps that, once taken, are followed by confirmation and blessing.

- **SHARE YOUR TRUTH.** Don't withhold wisdom or insight from others because of what they might think. Be what you believe, acting and speaking like God's ambassador wherever you go. When Dr. Taylor was a teenager, his dad would remind him as he left the house, *"Remember who you are and who you represent."*

- **LET GO OF THE OUTCOME.** How people perceive you, treat you, act or don't act on what you share, is up to them, not you. Your life is between you and God, not between you and them, and the same is true for anyone else. Trying to make everything OK with others will drag you, in the blink of an eye, into the cesspool that you just climbed out of, and that's no place for a child of God to live!

- **YOUR NEXT STEP:** You are not alone. Our mission is to deliver an easy to follow roadmap that supports your body, mind and spirit with direction, education and resources that you can easily master for life. We invite you to join our community of true health seekers who are creating lives of freedom, purpose, and joy. Learn more at www.WholeLifeWholeHealth.com.

"If you crave anything, you're missing something, and it's never what you crave."

Dr. Tom Taylor

Tools
for
Total Health

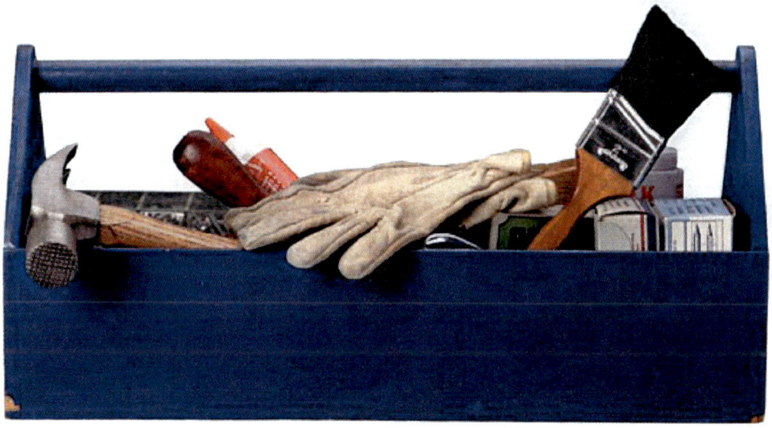

"We must understand that God's ultimate goal isn't healing. His goal is a body that has no sickness in it."

Cal Pierce, Director of The Healing Room Ministries
Spokane, Washington.

"Beloved, I pray that in all respects you may prosper and be in good health, just as your soul prospers."

The Apostle John, from 3 John 2, NASB

How To Cleanse For Maximum Success

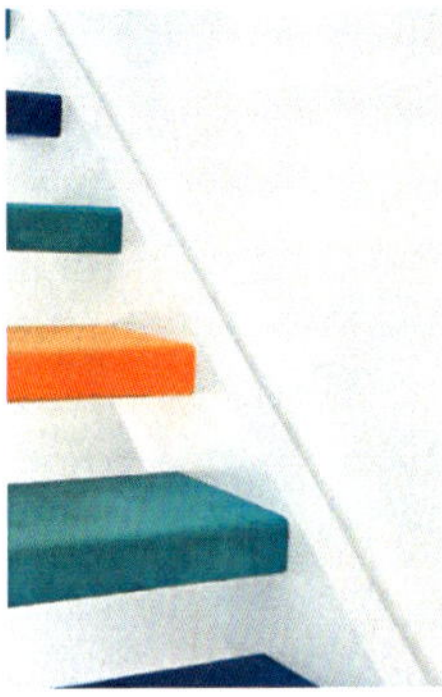

1. **Liver Rejuvenating Program** (pages 11-32) – Prepares the liver for efficient processing of toxins to be released in the cleanses that follow.

2. **Royal Flush®** (pages 33-38) – We highly recommend adding this on the third or fourth day after beginning to rejuvenate the liver, if bowels are moving properly. Stay on the **Royal Flush®** as long as it takes until your stool is normal. This can take months, but the results are worth it.

3. **4-Day Kidney, Liver and Gallbladder Cleanse** (pages 41-42) – Smoothes and flushes kidney stones painlessly, takes stress off these organs, enables better filtering and elimination of toxins in the blood stream, improves digestion of fats and absorption of fat-soluble vitamins, and helps restore the body's acid-alkaline balance.

   Although treated in modern medicine as a superfluous organ, the gallbladder is vital for regulating your body's all-important pH balance! This cleanse softens and rids cholesterol-based gallstones that you can't feel until it's too late. This powerful cleanse has saved many kidneys and gallbladders from surgery!

4. **10-Day Lemonade Cleanse** (page 49) – Now that the vital organs above can perform their functions efficiently, you're ready for a whole-body cellular cleanse. For at least 10 days, you'll be cleansing and rebuilding tissues and organs throughout your entire body.

- **The whole process is complete in less than a month.**
- **Repeat every six months to keep your insides squeaky clean.**
- **Check urine and saliva pH at the beginning and at the end.**

COMBINING CLEANSES FOR BEST RESULTS

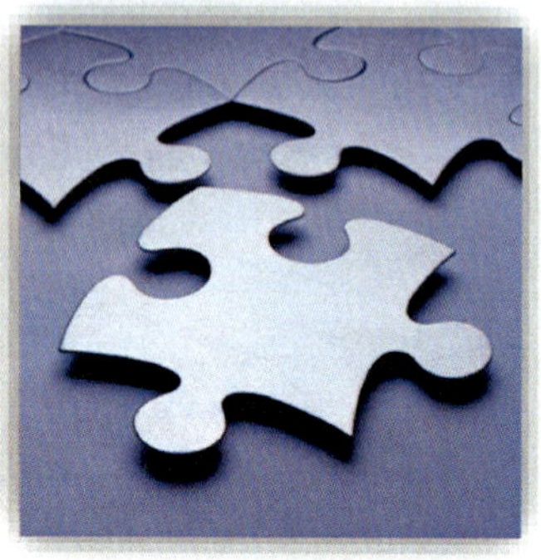

- **REJUVENATING THE LIVER** may be combined with the **ROYAL FLUSH®** and **SALTWATER FLUSH** (when necessary to help normalize the frequency of bowel movements). The dietary guidelines of **LIVER REJUVENATING** may be used at any time during, or apart from, other cleansing programs.

- The **ROYAL FLUSH®** may be used in combination with *any* other cleanse, including the **LEMONADE CLEANSE**.
    - Stop the **ROYAL FLUSH®** if bowels do not move at least 1-2 times per day. Begin the **SALTWATER FLUSH** immediately and continue until bowels move well and easily twice a day; then begin the **ROYAL FLUSH®** again.

- The **SALTWATER FLUSH** is highly desirable compared to laxatives or other stimulants. It may be used in combination with other cleanses to eliminate symptoms of toxin release, or any time bowels are sluggish.

- The **HEART, SOUL AND SPIRIT CLEANSE** is beneficial anytime and anywhere.

For more tips and information, log into YourPremiumWBC.wl-wh.com resource for True Health-Seekers.

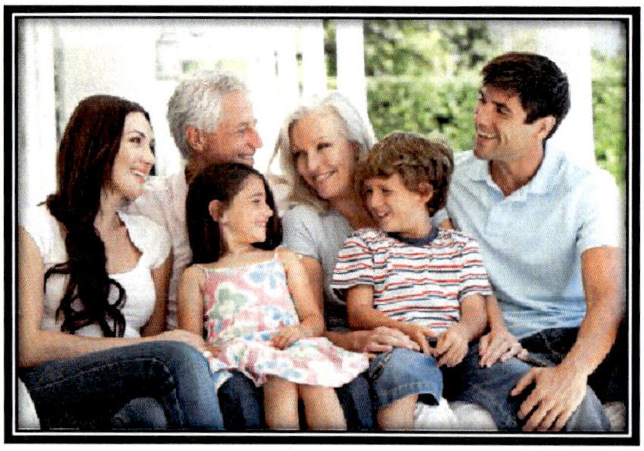

Positive Signs to Look For

Cleansing can reap tremendous benefits, and the list below shows just *some* that have been reported by clients. A few benefits may be experienced in days, while others may take weeks or even months to recognize, but be patient and persistent.

- ☐ General sense of well-being
- ☐ More alert
- ☐ More energy
- ☐ Improved elimination
- ☐ Improved digestion
- ☐ Improved appetite
- ☐ Improved sleep
- ☐ Need less sleep
- ☐ Wake up easier
- ☐ Wake up earlier
- ☐ Less urge to snack
- ☐ Less craving for sweets
- ☐ Increased desire for vegetables, salads
- ☐ Reduced weight
- ☐ Increased weight (some people want this!)
- ☐ Loss of size (waist, hips, neck, etc.)
- ☐ Improved skin tone/texture
- ☐ Improved visual acuity
- ☐ Improved sense of taste
- ☐ Nails grow stronger/faster
- ☐ Hair grows stronger/faster
- ☐ Look better
- ☐ Clearer eyes
- ☐ Easier to quit smoking
- ☐ Easier to exercise
- ☐ Easier to handle stress
- ☐ Faster recovery from exercise
- ☐ Able to work out harder
- ☐ Higher athletic performance
- ☐ Faster recovery from injury
- ☐ Reduced allergy symptoms
- ☐ Reduced sinus problems or colds
- ☐ Reduced arthritis symptoms
- ☐ Less pain overall
- ☐ Lower blood pressure
- ☐ Improved blood sugar balance
- ☐ Increased auditory sensitivity
- ☐ Improved breathing

The list above is not a guarantee of outcome. Individual results may vary widely.

In blood analysis of some clients, we often see improved cholesterol, signs of a higher functioning immune system, improved mineral reserves, and younger, healthier red blood cells that carry more oxygen everywhere!

As you follow ***Your Personal Roadmap to Whole Body Cleansing***, look for improvements in *every* facet of your life!

8 MASTER KEYS TO UNLOCK YOUR TOTAL HEALTH

Bodies respond perfectly, for the purpose of survival, to the choices *we* make in eight areas:

1. **What you EAT**
2. **What you DRINK**
3. **What and How you BREATHE**
4. **How you EXERCISE (or don't)**
5. **How you REST**
6. **What you THINK, FEEL and BELIEVE**
7. **What you SPEAK**
8. **How you NURTURE your SPIRIT**

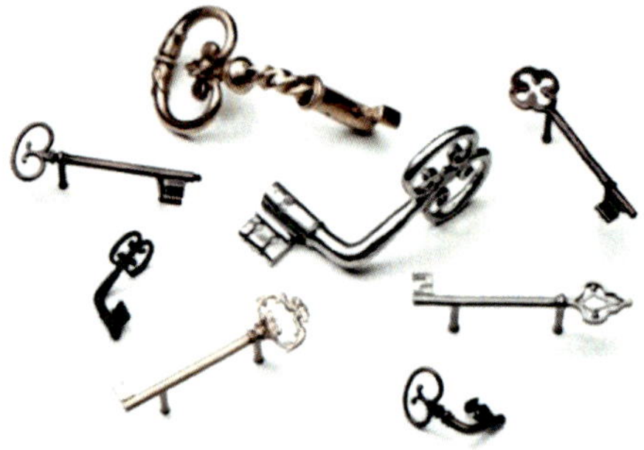

The better choices you make, the better your body works and the better you feel. It's just that simple.

The following is a brief discussion of each of the eight areas in which we're in total charge; it is by no means complete! For more information about these areas, go to www.8keys.wholelifewholehealth.com.

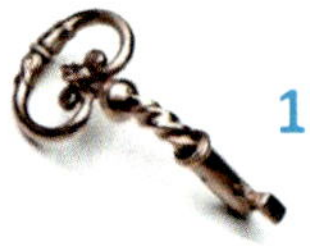

1. **WHAT YOU EAT:** This subject is so controversial, yet so simple that almost no one believes it. Ready?

- 75% vegetables and fruit (organically grown is best); at least half of those should be raw.
- 25% nuts, seeds, grains, dairy, and flesh (anything with eyes) – in that order.
- Fill your plate with the brightest and deepest colors, because they are the most nutrient-dense foods.

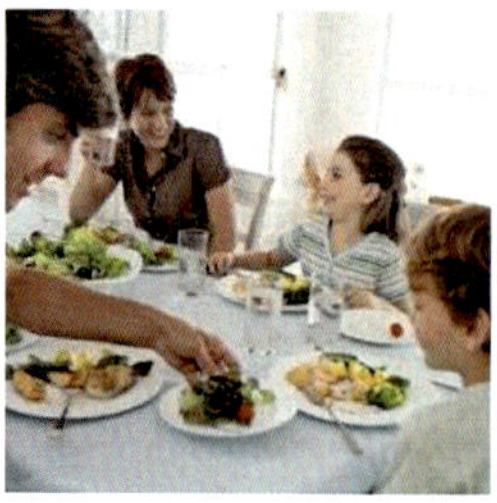

2. **WHAT YOU DRINK:** This subject is also somewhat controversial, but it's even simpler...**WATER**! We're made mostly of 75-85 percent water, depending on what authority you check. Here are the water sources we recommend, in the order we recommend them:

- ALKALINE IONIZED WATER (see page 63-64)
- **Reverse Osmosis (RO) Water**
- **Activated Carbon Filtered Water**
- **Spring Water**
- **Tap Water**

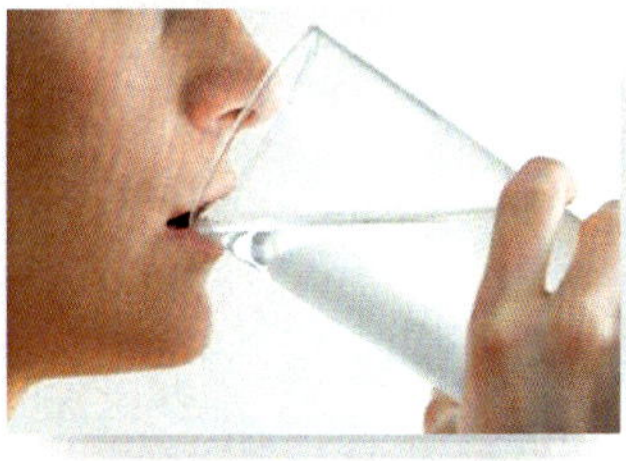

3. **WHAT YOU BREATHE:** If you can see the air, you're in trouble (fog doesn't count). If the air around you smells, and the smell is manmade, i.e. chemical, open a window or filter the air. Obviously, smoking is out.

HOW YOU BREATHE: This should be simple enough; breathe in, breathe out; what's the big deal? Look at a baby breathe. Their little bellies expand and contract like little balloons, but their chests stay fairly still. Compare that with how you normally breathe; almost the opposite, right?

Babies know how to breathe correctly, because they're totally at peace; they aren't in emergency mode, "running from bears." You need to remember how to breathe like that too. When you do, you'll find you're less stressed and more peaceful, no matter what's going on around you.

BELLY BREATHING: Breathe into your belly; hold it in; breathe out; hold it out. Perform each step to a slow count of four. Repeat the cycle at least four times. That's it: 4 steps, to a 4 count, 4 times.*

*Go to **YourPremiumWBC.wl-wh.com** for a special downloadable "cheat sheet."

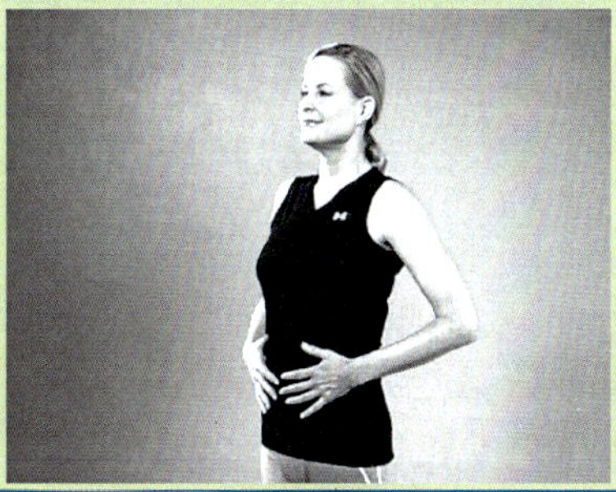

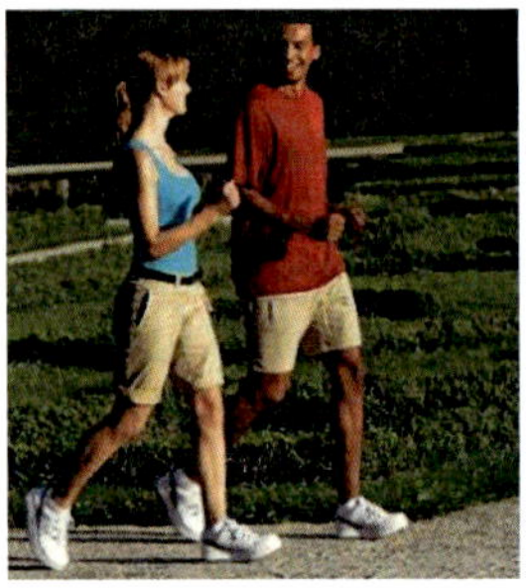

4. **HOW YOU EXERCISE (or don't):** The most natural exercise is walking. It's what you grew up with; it doesn't take any special skills or expensive equipment, and you can do it around your own neighborhood. Check out this web site for great information on how to begin a walking program: TheWalkingSite.com.

In addition to walking, we teach clients and workshop audiences the **VICTORY MARCH**, a combination of Yoga, Tai-Chi, Qigong, and controlled breathing. It's a free neurological upgrade, improving flexibility, balance, coordination, stamina, and even temperament, all in 28 days. The movement is a hugely exaggerated walk, which can be performed in a few square feet. Download an instruction sheet of how to perform the **VICTORY MARCH** for maximum benefit on YourPremiumWBC.wl-wh.com.

Here's an idea of what the VICTORY MARCH looks like and how it works:

- The stance is a bit like a lunge. Be sure to keep your front knee bent and your back knee straight, with both heels planted.
- This is a "cross-crawl" stance, so the arm opposite to the front knee is raised, while the other arm points straight back.
- Look over the shoulder of the raised arm, as far as you can turn your head without straining; look up diagonally with your eyes.
- Close your eyes, take in a breath, and hold this position (eyes closed) for as long as you can, or for a count of 10.
- Exhale, open your eyes, and switch legs, arms, and head position.
- Repeat this procedure back and forth, from side to side, for four complete cycles.

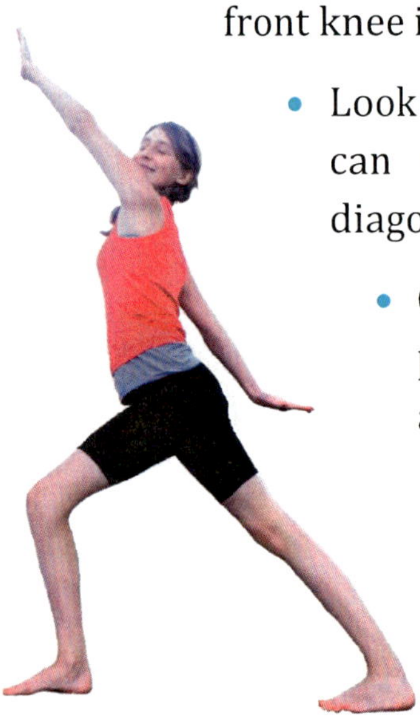

5. **HOW YOU REST:** Rest and sleep aren't necessarily the same. If sleep isn't restful, you don't feel well; you don't perform well; and you may be tough to live with.

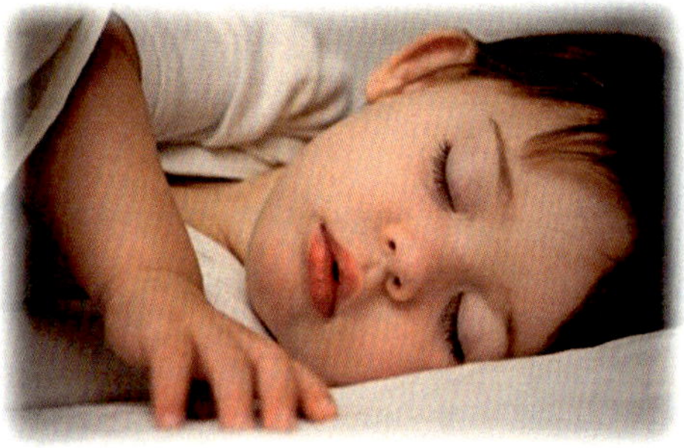

Although there is some agreement that adults need seven to nine hours of sleep per night, authorities note that the number of hours of sleep needed varies from person to person. Agreement is unanimous, however, that *restful* sleep, whatever the number of hours, is essential to physical and mental health and well-being.

TWO SIMPLE RULES OF RESTFUL SLEEP:

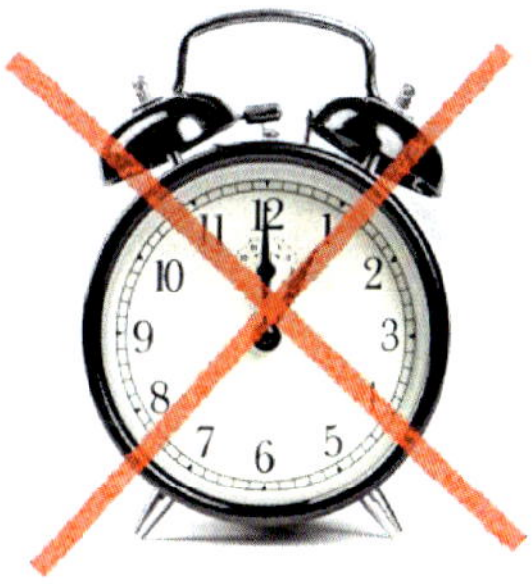

1. If you need an alarm clock to wake up, you need to go to bed earlier. Yes, we know that may not be easy, but we also know it can be done, and waking up naturally – free of alarms – is certainly more peaceful, and it may even make the rest of the day less stressful overall. An exception to the "no alarm clock" rule is one with a light that brightens gradually, to simulate a sunrise.

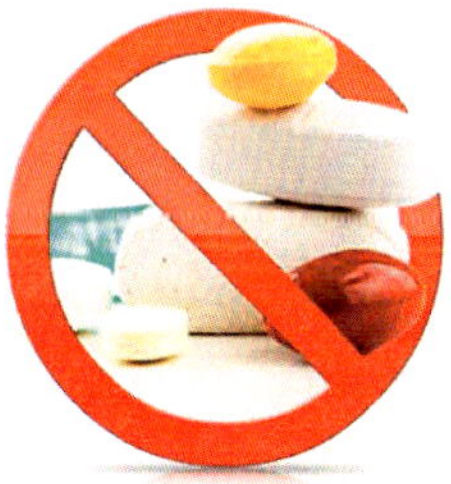

2. If you take a drug or use a device to help you sleep, an underlying problem – an unanswered alarm – needs to be addressed. Work with a holistic health practitioner and use the **HEART, SOUL AND SPIRIT CLEANSE**.

6. **WHAT YOU THINK, FEEL AND BELIEVE:** You've probably heard phrases like, "Thoughts are things," and, "What you believe you become." The spirit-mind-body connection is real; you're operating it all the time, whether you know it or not, like it or not, or believe it or not; and it's more important than all of the preceding keys combined.

> ***"For as he thinks within himself so he is."***
>
> (Proverbs 23:7, NASB)

In 1990, my earliest mentor in this field showed me how my physical body was directly connected to – and would make instantaneous changes according to – my thoughts, feelings, and beliefs. The simple "muscle test" he performed was so astonishing that I made him repeat it several times. Suddenly, a new awareness dawned and it has never left: My physical, mental, emotional, and spiritual well-being affects every area of my life and is entirely up to me. I also realized that if this was true for me, then it was true for everyone around me.

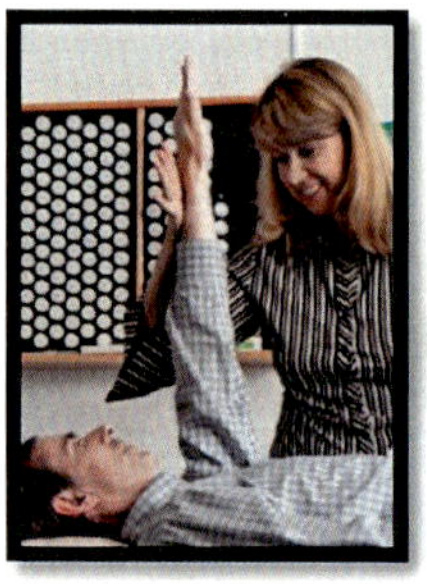

The implications were staggering – they still are – and we have seen them play out in thousands of lives, in countless conditions (physical, financial, relational...you name it):

> **You determine how sick or healthy you are – not genes, not family history – *YOU* do it and you can also undo it. Your thoughts, feelings, beliefs, and the habits they produce, determine your well-being in every area of life.**

This key, quite literally, is the heart and soul of the **HEART, SOUL AND SPIRIT CLEANSE**, on pages 70-82. Master these steps, along with the other keys, and you have the best opportunity to walk in divine health, flying through any limitation, and living the victory!

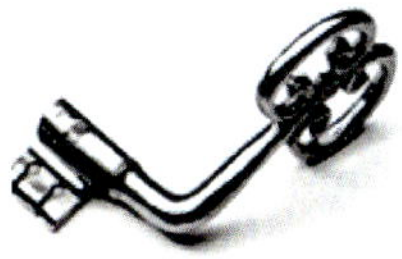

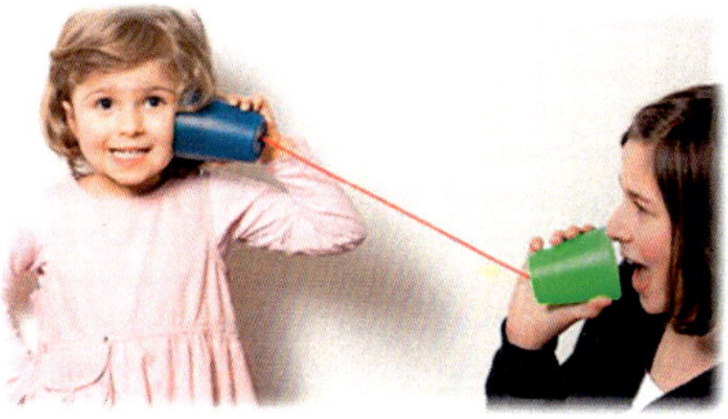

7. **WHAT YOU SPEAK:** The simple truth is, ***"out of the super-abundance of the heart the mouth is speaking"*** (Matthew 12:34).

Speech – your language – is a way of communicating, but the question is, what are you communicating? What you speak has the power to create or destroy, bless or curse, encourage or criticize…yourself and others. We have heard countless people claim their illness, i.e., *"My Diabetes," "My depression,"* or *"My cancer."* How many times have you heard someone say, *"I can't…," "I don't think I'll ever…," "You can't…," or, "You'll never…"?* Words not only express, but can also affect what you think, feel, and believe.

Speaking also involves hearing, so whatever you speak comes right back to you!

Words both reflect and affect what you think, feel, and believe.

Charles Capps' book, ***The Tongue: A Creative Force***, is one of the most helpful resources we've found to help understand the power of our words. Capps writes, *"[People] can have what they say, [but instead] they are saying what they have."*

You are probably familiar with "affirmations," and we enjoy being around people who celebrate life in every area. We observe, however, that most people talk about – they affirm – what they don't like, don't want, or don't have. Affirmations work both ways, so ask yourself what your affirmations sound like; are you celebrating or complaining?

"From the fruit of a man's mouth his stomach will be satisfied; He will be satisfied with the product of his lips. Death and life lie in the power of the tongue, and those who love it will eat its fruit." **(Proverbs 18:20-21, NASB)**

8. **HOW YOU NURTURE YOUR SPIRIT:** Dancing delicately around the spirit of the **HEART, SOUL AND SPIRIT CLEANSE** is a waste of valuable time, so let's dive into the deep end together and learn to swim.

> **You are a spiritual being undergoing a physical experience, not the other way around.**

I was taught that the nervous system controlled and directed every function of the human body, but I'm persuaded that the spirit animates life itself, directs all functions that the nervous system only carries out, and enables healing to take place. People who are strong and actively aware in their spirits are usually also aware and active in their healing process. They develop a militant posture toward protecting themselves from pain and illness by establishing habits that support, rather than undermine health and well-being. They develop a highly tuned inner sense of "hearing" and, when alarm bells sound inside *(see page 71)*, often before pain, illness, tragedy, or even lack threatens, they look immediately for the cause, address it, and thereby make suffering unnecessary to continue, worsen, or to recur.

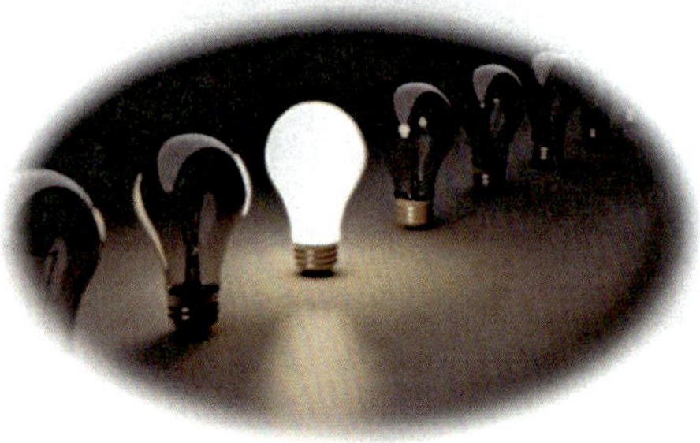

The Spirit of God, which gives life, instills your spirit to sustain it, and it goes back to God at the end of life. It's that simple. Scientists and other experts in human energy fields and quantum physics, recognize the presence of your spirit. They use terms like "energy field," "information field," or "innate intelligence," but behind the words is the inescapable, intangible spirit.

> ***"The dust returns to the ground it came from, and the spirit returns to God Who gave it."***
> (Ecclesiastes 12:7)

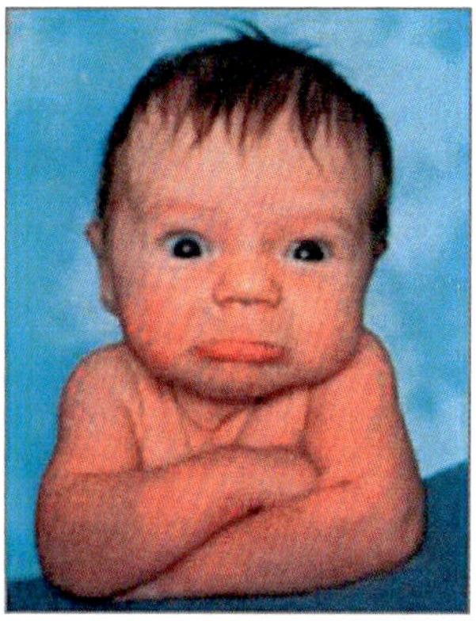

Your spirit takes the first hit of any insult and sounds the first alarms, whether the insult comes through the five senses or through your own thoughts, feelings and beliefs about your experiences and relationships. The physical body is the last in line to feel the effects of an insult, but it is usually the first in line to get your attention. The longer the alarm has been sounding, the more symptoms there are, the worse they are, and/or the more life-threatening and urgent they become.

The HEART, SOUL AND SPIRIT CLEANSE *(pages 70-82)* was developed as a consistently reliable way to move through an acute crisis or a chronic situation successfully. It is simply the fastest, most direct way we have found to identify the landmarks that limit healing, performance, advancement, or fulfillment, and break through to the "other side," where you are living free and living in victory.

Whatever you believe, no one healed like Jesus. The best examples of rapid, lasting healing are found throughout the life of Jesus Christ and the apostles who followed after Him. If Jesus were standing beside you right now, you would know that healing was only a word or touch away.

What condition are you in today? If any area of life is less than joyfully, abundantly and purposefully healthy, consider inviting the Spirit of God and the life of Jesus Christ into yours. If you are already familiar with the life of God's Spirit operating in your own spirit, you may need to increase your intimacy with it; if not, you can become acquainted with it.

The *ALKALINE TRACKER*™

How to Track and Score Your Diet For Maximum Health

All of the cleansing programs in the previous pages enable the body to achieve acid-alkaline balance as discussed on pages 57-66. The ***ALKALINE TRACKER***™ was designed to help you track your daily diet by scoring what you eat and drink on a simple scale to show you how close you are to achieving an alkaline body chemistry.

HERE'S HOW IT WORKS:

1. List what you eat and drink at each meal, as well as any snacks. Be honest – it's only your health!
2. Assign a simple score for each food:

   -1 for acid-producing foods

   +1 for alkaline-producing foods

> **Go to**
> **YOURPREMIUMWBC.WL-WH.COM**
> **for acid-alkaline food charts.**

3. Add the number of acid and alkaline foods, and arrive at a total for the day. You'll quickly see how well you're doing by the end of each week! You may also be surprised at what it takes to have an alkaline body!

Three Simple Rules to Remember

- Animal protein is acid-forming.
- Nuts (except almonds and Brazil nuts), seeds and grains (except millet and quinoa), are acid-forming.
- All vegetables and most fruits are alkaline-producing.

Follow the sample *ALKALINE TRACKER*™ on the following page . . .

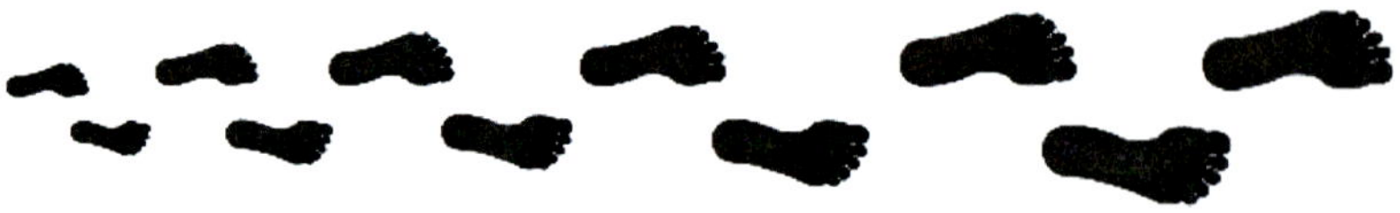

SAMPLE *ALKALINE TRACKER™*

Alkaline Foods are shaded

Meal	Mon.			Thurs.			
Breakfast	Orange Juice Toast w/ Butter 2 eggs Coffee	+1 -1 -2 -1	**Each egg counts!**	Royal Flush® 2 Juice Plus+® Fruit caps and 1 Berry cap.	+2 +3	**Each drink & each capsule counts!**	
Lunch	Tuna Salad Sandwich Potato Chips Apple	-2 -1 +1	**Tuna and bread each count as one!**	Big Salad w/ Almonds Hummus on Crisp-bread	+2 +1 +1 -1		
Dinner	Green Beans Salad Chicken Coffee	+1 +1 -1 -1	**BIG salads could count as 2! Each piece of Chicken counts!**	Power Shake Almond Butter w/apple 2 JP+® veggie caps, 1 Berry cap.	0 +1 +1 +3	**The shake is neutral**	
Snacks	Apple Coffee Cookies Pop Corn	+1 -1 -1 -1	**Coffee and Tea count!**	Water-melon Crisp bread w/Boursin cheese & sprouts	+1 -1 -1 +1		
Acid (-1)	-12			-3			
Alkaline (+1)	+5			+16			
TOTAL SCORE	**-7**			**+13**			

Copy this **Alkaline Tracker**™ for your own use!

MY *ALKALINE TRACKER*™

Meal	Mon.	Tues.	Weds.	Thurs.	Fri.	Sat.	Sun.
Breakfast							
Lunch							
Dinner							
Snacks							
Acid (-1)							
Alkaline (+1)							
TOTAL SCORE							

MIRACLES WITH MINERALS

Your body functions according to God's design, not your desire. The natural order works only one way:

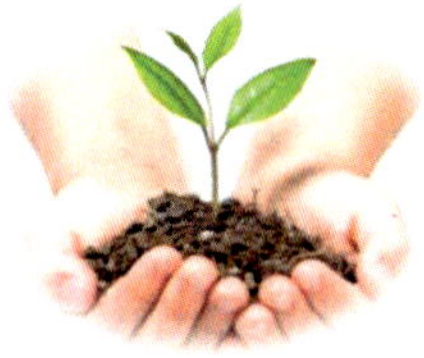

- **The Mineral kingdom feeds the Plant kingdom**
  - Plants derive minerals from the soil
- **The Plant kingdom feeds the Animal kingdom**
  - Animals derive minerals from plant foods
  - Animals cannot derive usable minerals directly from the soil

Minerals are miraculous molecules, essential to facilitate more than 10,000 chemical reactions taking place each second in every one of trillions of cells that make up your body's tissues, organs and systems.

"Macro minerals" are required in relatively large amounts (over 100mg), and include sodium, potassium, magnesium, calcium, phosphorus, and chloride. "Trace minerals" (also called "trace elements") are required in tiny amounts, many of them more than 1,000 times less than macro minerals. Of the dozens of trace minerals, ones that are commonly recognized include zinc, iron, copper, iodine, and manganese.

Our soil has been depleted of many minerals since the advent of modern farming in the early 1900s. Even a diet rich in organically grown vegetables and fruit is deficient in minerals. A mineral supplement has become a basic daily requirement for disease prevention, and long-term health and well-being.

Sagging skin, wrinkles, premature aging, poor sleep, memory loss, and hormonal imbalance, are some of the landmarks of mineral deficiency.

The best mineral supplement will be derived from plant materials, which have broken down the inorganic material from the soil and rock into minute particles that are usable. The best supplement is a liquid in which these microscopic particles are suspended in a solution high in fulvic acid.

We use TRACE MINERALS PLUS+® from an ancient plant deposit of "humic shale." Over millions of years, plant material is compressed into layers that look like coal. Once extracted from the earthen deposit, the mineral substance is allowed to sit in the sun and air for about a year, until it becomes a sandy consistency. Water is dripped slowly through the "sand," and the result is a "colloid," rich in fulvic acid, in which mineral particles are so small they can be absorbed and utilized by your body.

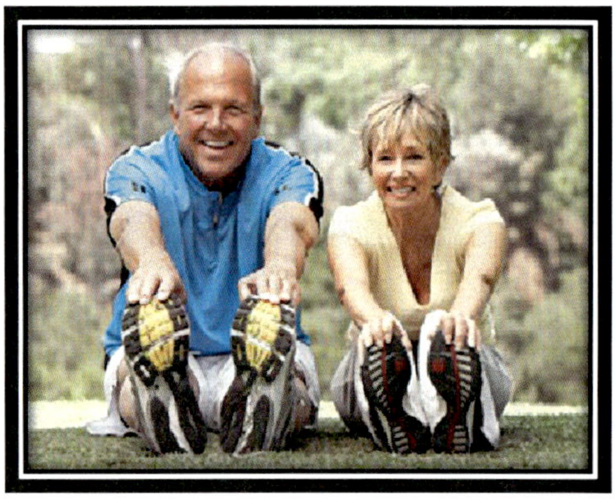

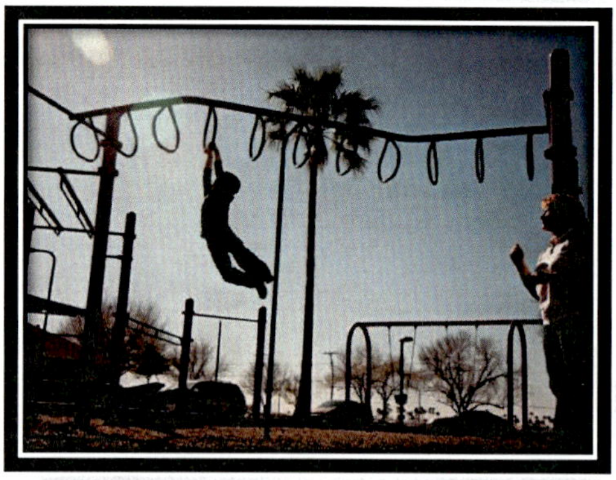

Every "medicine cabinet," purse, briefcase, office desk, glove compartment, gym bag, suitcase, and First Aid Kit should have a bottle of TRACE MINERALS PLUS+®!

Important Points About Liquid Minerals

- **Liquid minerals stain!**

  If the liquid gets on fabric, use a spot remover and wash it right away. With some fabrics, this may not even work. It's best to keep everything away from liquid minerals except what you want them on!

- **Never heat liquid minerals!**

  Heat kills the vital properties of liquid minerals; however, a few drops in bath water can help neutralize the chlorine in tap water.

- **Liquid minerals are highly astringent.**

  Never use them directly in the eyes! If exposure occurs, flush with water immediately.

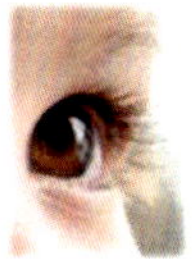

- **Liquid minerals are super bitter!**

  We've never chewed on a rusty nail, but that's the image that comes to mind. Put a drop on your tongue, if you'd like to gain first-hand experience of the unique, incredibly bitter taste of liquid minerals.

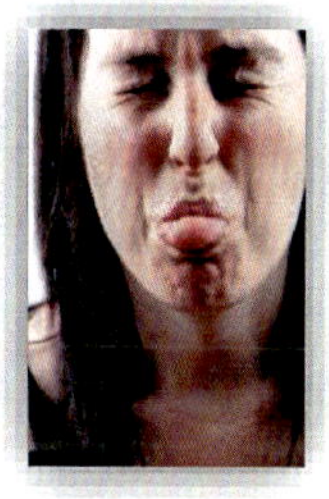

- **Liquid minerals can sting.**

  When applying liquid minerals to open wounds, especially for kids and animals, mix 1 drop of minerals with 2-4 drops of water.

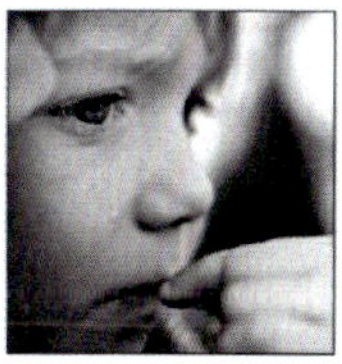

- **No "bad guy bugs" can live with liquid minerals.**

  Liquid minerals naturally kill and repel unfriendly bacteria and viruses, but they'll never hurt you when used properly.

First Aid With Trace Minerals Plus+®

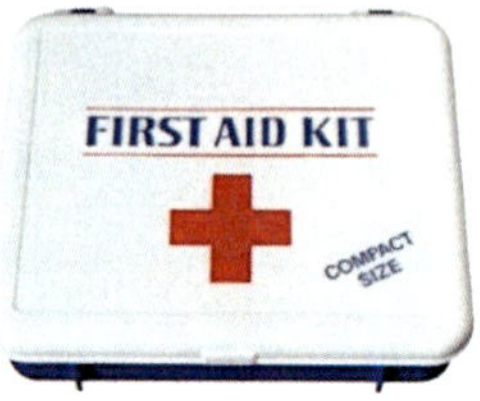

Trace Minerals Plus+® has tremendous healing properties that we have been privileged to experience firsthand and witness in the lives of countless individuals and families since the early 1990's.

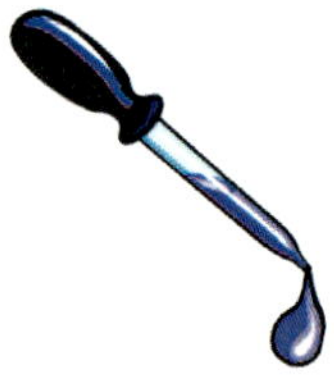

The following are some of the most common applications for which **Trace Minerals Plus+®** has proven to deliver effective first aid.

- **CUTS**

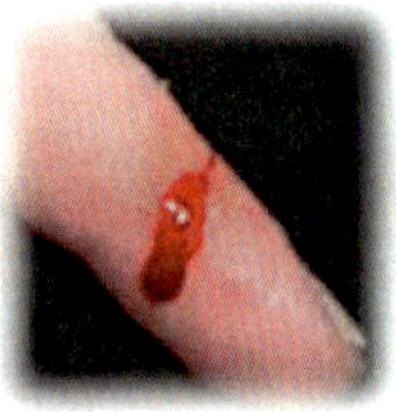

After cleaning a wound, put a drop of **Trace Minerals Plus+®** (or more, depending on wound size) directly on the cut or wound. This will most often cauterize the bleeding. Deeper wounds may require bandaging and pressure, but **Trace Minerals Plus+®** will help cauterize and disinfect the wound until medical attention can be obtained.

- **BURNS**

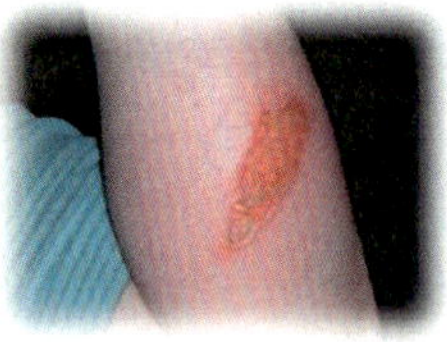

Put **Trace Minerals Plus+®** on any burn area, followed by ice. Do this twice. Often, after the second application of minerals and ice, no blister will raise and often you won't even be able to find the burn!

- **SORE THROATS**

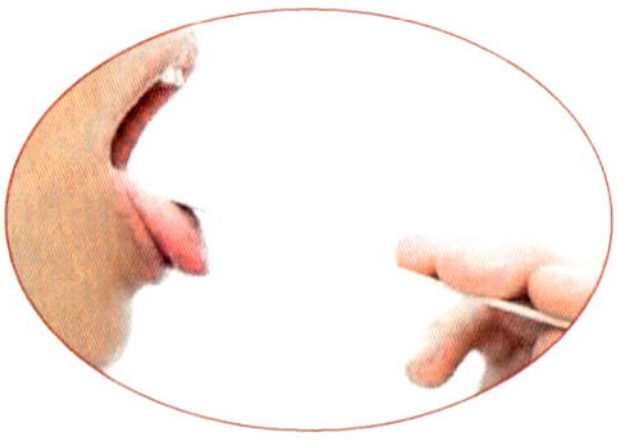

Put 4-5 drops of **Trace Minerals Plus+®** in 1-2 oz. of water, gargle and swallow. Once may be enough if you catch it early. If not, repeat 3-6 times per day. The condition should clear up in 1-2 days (even Thrush and Strep Throat).

- **SINUS INFECTIONS**

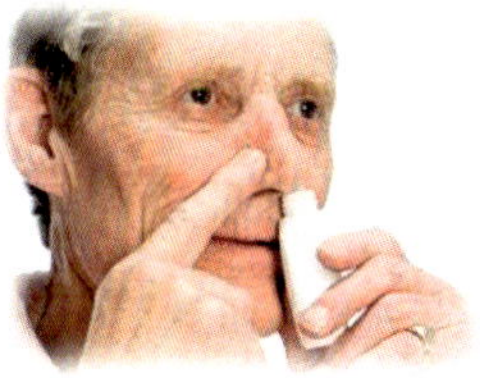

Put 4-6 drops of **TRACE MINERALS PLUS+®** in an ounce of saline solution (salt water) from any drugstore, with a cap that allows you to create a nasal spray. Spray and inhale the mixture through each nostril into the sinuses. Get tissues ready, because the sludge that you'll blow out is unbelievable! For impacted sinuses, more than one application may be needed, but they'll often clear within 24 hours. This method works for sinus congestion too!

- **BOILS, SKIN ERUPTIONS**

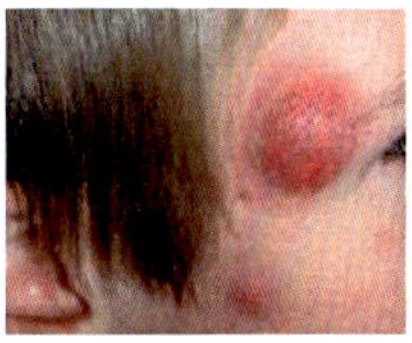

Use like you would for cuts and wounds. Wet a bandage pad with 2-3 drops of **TRACE MINERALS PLUS+®** and cover the area. Do this twice a day for as long as needed. Boils usually clear up in a few days.

- **TOOTH ABSCESSES** (or impacted teeth)

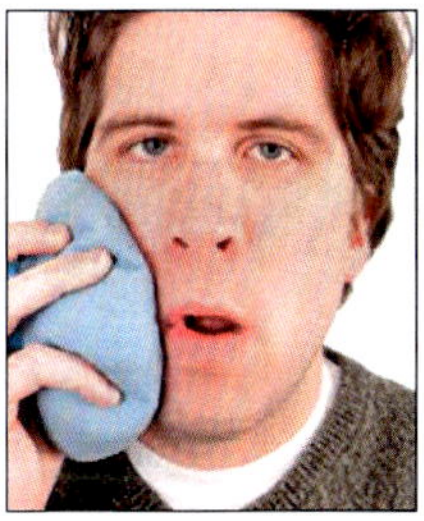

Soak Q-Tip™ with 3-4 drops of **TRACE MINERALS PLUS+®** and rub into the gum line at the involved tooth *(Note: You will taste the minerals)*. Repeat this a few times a day until you can get to your dentist, or until the abscess clears or resolves itself; but don't wait more than a couple of days.

  - **ADDITIONAL HELP:** After applying **TRACE MINERALS PLUS+®**, open a capsule of probiotics and massage into the gum line.

- **COLD AND CHANCRE SORES**

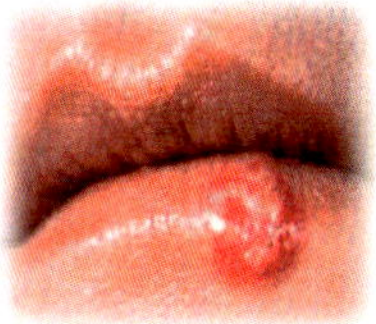

Apply 1 drop of **TRACE MINERALS PLUS+®** directly to the area. Use a Q-Tip™ if you like. Liquid minerals will stain external sores, but they can clear up in less than 24 hours. For internal sores, use as described for tooth remedies above and repeat as needed.

- **INTERNAL BLEEDING**

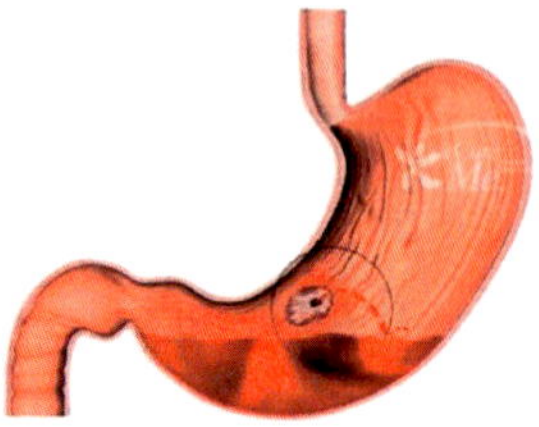

Mix 1 teaspoon of **TRACE MINERALS PLUS+®** in orange or grapefruit juice, and drink daily for 3 days. If the stool turns black, continue for 21 days. Stool should change to brown within that time. If not, seek medical help.

- **SUNBURN**

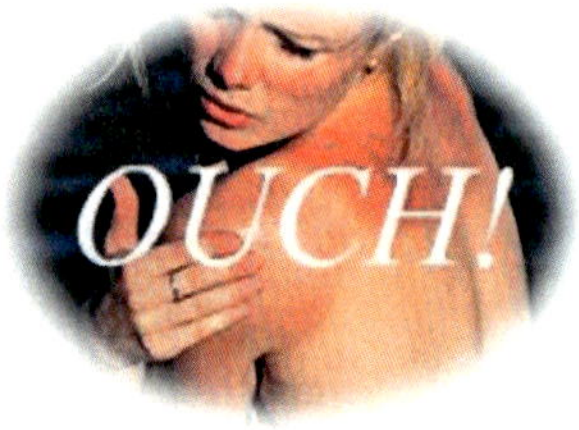

Apply **TRACE MINERALS PLUS+®** directly to the sunburned area (use a soaked cotton pad). If the area is quite large, put 1 tablespoon of **TRACE MINERALS PLUS+®** in a tub of water that is just warm enough to get in, and bathe for 10-20 minutes. You may need to repeat this daily until the burn heals, depending on its severity.

- **HEMORRHOIDS**

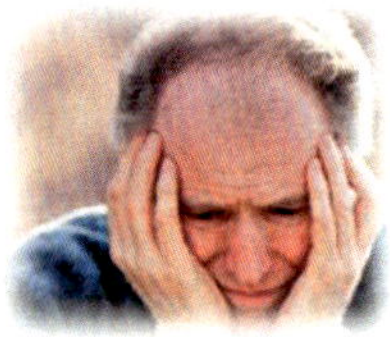

If hemorrhoids aren't bleeding, put 3-4 drops of **TRACE MINERALS PLUS+®** on a single square of toilet paper folded in quarters. Apply the minerals directly on the hemorrhoids with pressure; then apply ointment over the area (our favorite is "Neem" ointment). For bleeding hemorrhoids, make a "sitz bath" of warm water and a teaspoon of **TRACE MINERALS PLUS+®**. Sit in the solution for at least 5 minutes and repeat twice daily until tissues heal enough to apply the minerals directly, (usually 1-2 days).

- **SYSTEMIC YEAST INFECTIONS (Candida)**

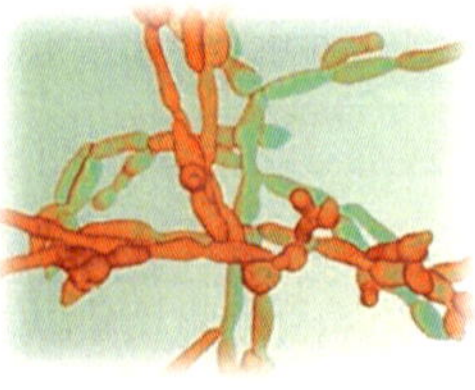

Use ¼ teaspoon of **TRACE MINERALS PLUS+®** 3 times per day in water (remember, this tastes bitter). Avoid *ALL* dairy, grains, refined sugar, and fruit. This can take several weeks to clear up.

- **VAGINAL YEAST AND VAGINITIS**

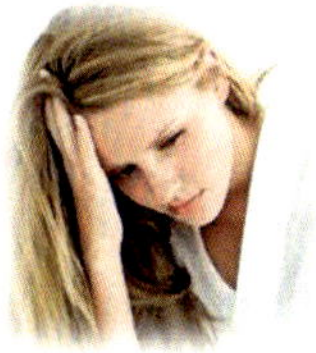

Prepare a douche container filled with sterile saline. Add 4 drops of **TRACE MINERALS PLUS+®** and apply 1-2 times per day. This will often clear up even the most raging infection in 1-3 days.

- **EAR INFECTIONS**

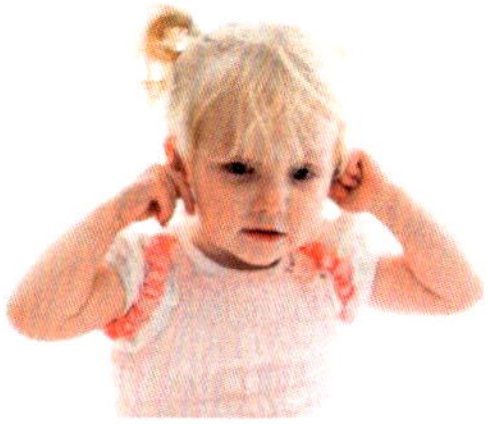

Put 1-2 drops of **TRACE MINERALS PLUS+®** directly into the affected ear, pack gently with cotton, and apply moist heat (hot water bottles work well), while lying on the affected side. Repeat 2-3 times a day. Infections often clear in a day or less.

- **TRAVELING**

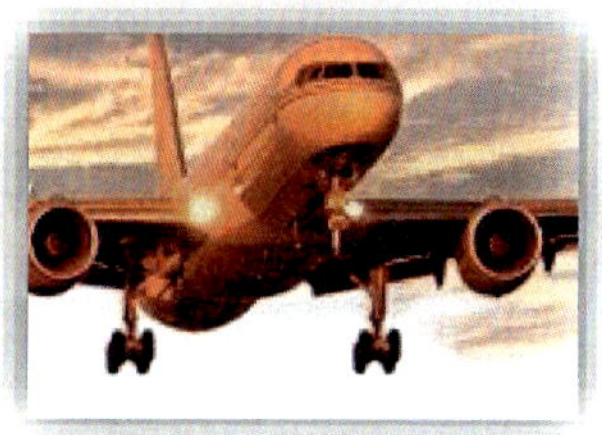

Take *at least* a teaspoon of **TRACE MINERALS PLUS+®** per day when traveling to avoid diarrhea from unfamiliar water and foods.

Blast Colds, Flu and Allergies With Nutrition!

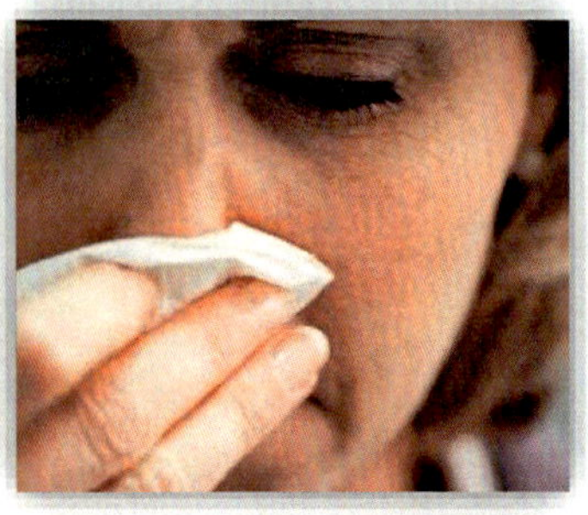

We view colds, flu, and allergies as natural cleansing processes that your body resorts to at a time when your immune system is challenged beyond its normal limits, by exposure to other sick people, unfamiliar or excess toxins, seasonal changes, or even mental and emotional stress.

Colds tend to affect mucous membranes in the sinuses and lungs, while influenza affects the joints. Allergies may affect all of these in addition to the eyes and mouth.

GAME PLAN FOR COLDS AND FLU:

- **Take 30-50mg high-quality Zinc with 3** DAILY ENZYME COMPLEX **three times per day until symptoms clear** (this should only take 1-3 days).
- **Then take the same regimen twice a day for 3-5 more days, and at the first sign of any more symptoms.**
- **Add Airborne® to the regimen for an extra boost and to further shorten the duration and severity of symptoms.**
- **If symptoms don't clear up within 2 days, add 3 probiotic capsules between meals.**

IMPORTANT:

Avoid *ALL* dairy products, fruit or fruit juices, especially citrus juices, and most especially, orange juice! Fruits are cleansing and oranges have a sulphur-containing protein. *Bottom line:* These foods make symptoms worse and last longer.

ALLERGIES

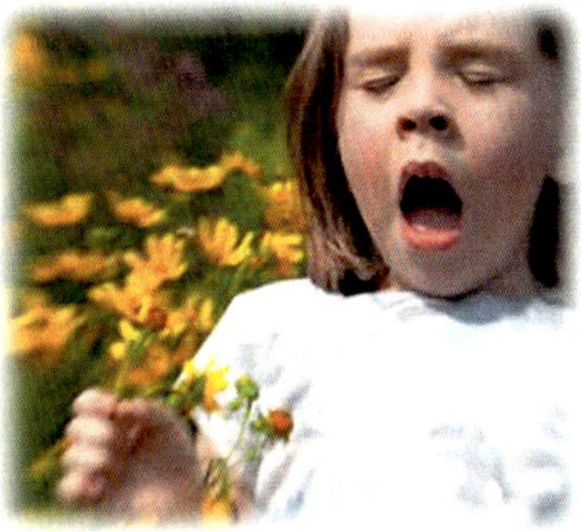

We find that allergens (substances that "*cause*" allergy symptoms) are, for the most part, incompletely processed or digested particles on top of many others.

You tend to challenge your body's reserves in the first place, by what you eat, drink and think; when seasons change or you encounter unfamiliar foods or toxins, your already maxed-out immune systems throw a "histamine fit." All this is an inflammation response, while your body attempts to rid the excess load through your mucus membranes or your skin. Anyone with allergies knows the result: itchy mouth, itchy or teary eyes, congestion, coughing, sneezing, headaches, loose stools, and even rashes.

ALLERGY GAME PLAN:

- **Take 1 Airborne® tablet in water with 3 DAILY ENZYME COMPLEX.**
- **Repeat every 3 hours until symptoms disappear** (should only take a few doses).
- **Then take the same regimen twice a day for 3-5 more days and at the first sign of any more symptoms.**
- **If symptoms don't clear up within 2 days, add 3 probiotic capsules between meals, or more to resolve symptoms.**

IMPORTANT:

Just like for colds and flu, avoid *ALL* dairy products, fruit or fruit juices, especially citrus juices, and most especially, orange juice! Fruits are cleansing and oranges have a sulphur-containing protein. *Bottom line:* These foods make symptoms worse and last longer.

HOME REMEDIES TRIED AND TRUE

- **Soothe & Silence Ear Aches**

  Put 2-3 drops of **warm garlic oil** in the ear canal and follow other instructions on page 119. Repeat several times a day if needed.

- **Stop Gallbladder Attack Fast**

  Drink 1 tablespoon of non-distilled **apple cider vinegar** in a glass of apple juice.

- **No More Jet Lag**

  Put a few drops of **lavender essential oil** (pharmaceutical grade) on the hands or wrists and breathe the scent periodically throughout long flights. This has virtually eliminated jet lag even for huge time differences!

- **Calm Stress/Anxiety/Moods**

  1-2 drops of a Bach® Flower Remedy, called **Rescue® Remedy**.

- **Silence Night Time Coughs**

  At bedtime, apply olive oil with a few drops of **essential oil (peppermint or eucalyptus)** or **Vick's Vapo-Rub®** to the soles of your feet and put on socks. No coughing. No kidding!

- **Relax Muscles Naturally**

  Take 1-3 tablets of **FORMULA 303®**, a blend of Valerian Root, Passion Flower and Magnesium. It relaxes without making you drowsy or loopy, like drugs.

- **Sleep Like a Baby**

  Combine 1 tablet of **FORMULA 303®** before bed time with calcium and **CORTISOLV®**.

- **Quick Fix for Inflammation**

  Zyflamend® is an herbal product that often gets results that are as good or better than drugs, without the side effects! Follow the label directions.

- **Heal Raw Skin, Diaper Rash**

  Neem cream has an amazing ability to heal some of the worst raw skin conditions we've seen, and it works fast! Neem may be applied as often as needed.

- **Stop or Reduce Bruising**

  Arnica gel applied ASAP to a bruised area will often prevent or reduce discoloration. **Arnica gel** also helps relieve sore or strained muscles, and sprained joints.

The Weight is Over

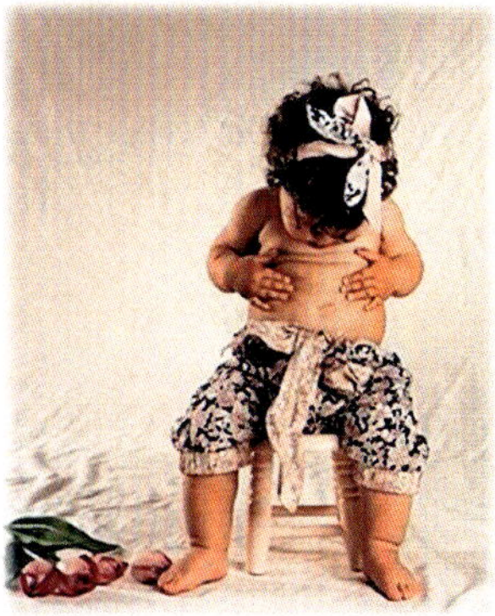

We prefer *eliminating* rather than merely *losing* excess weight. Many people lose weight only to find it again, and add even more! The weight-loss industry is enormous, and there are programs a-plenty from which to choose. You've probably tried some already!

Eliminating excess weight naturally accompanies effective cleansing processes.

As the body sheds stored toxins and the water needed to dilute them, becoming cleaner and healthier all the time, extra "insulation" is no longer needed, so it's eliminated. The body is able to release even "stubborn" excess weight naturally. There's no guarantee, however, that you'll achieve your ideal shape and size after going through the cleanses in the proper order only once *(see page 99)*.

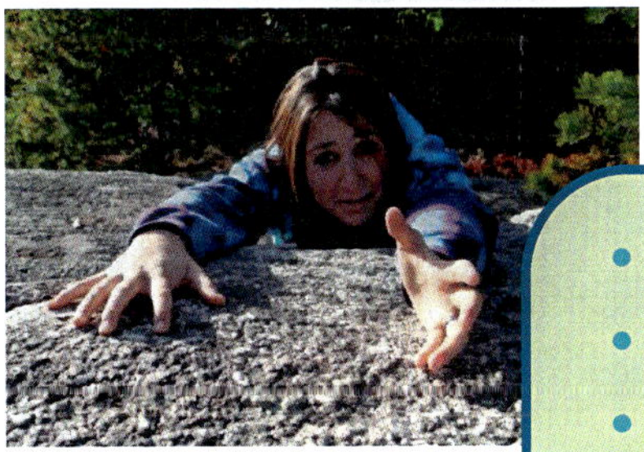

KITCHEN COMBAT

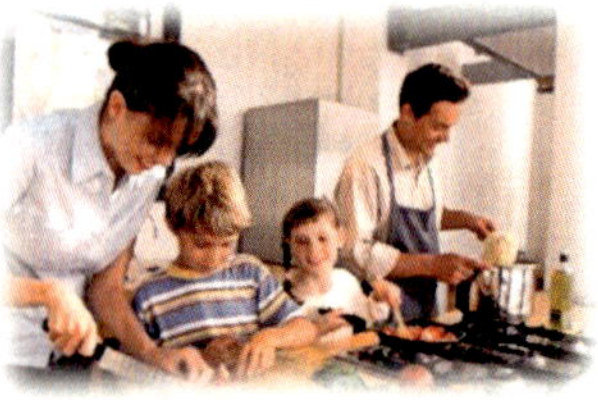

You want to make a healthy meal, but the kitchen might feel like a combat zone, with all manner of sharp instruments, fire, and perhaps a family daring you to come up with something "good" for dinner.

These are just a few essentials to have on hand at all times, ready to mix and match whenever a creative spark begins. The lists below are by no means complete; add to them to suit your and your family's needs.

BASIC EQUIPMENT

- ✓ Blender
- ✓ Food Processor
- ✓ Mixer (hand-held)
- ✓ Convection Oven
- ✓ Wok – stainless steel that requires "seasoning"
- ✓ Pepper Mill
- ✓ Garlic Press
- ✓ Knives (Paring, Carving, Cleaver, Bread, smooth & serrated)
- ✓ Knife Sharpener

BASIC PANTRY

✓ **OILS**
- Cold-Pressed, Extra Virgin Olive Oil
- Sesame
- Coconut
- Butter

✓ **SPICES**
- Sea Salt
- Pepper, whole, black & white
- Paprika
- Tamari or Teriyaki

✓ **HERBS**
- Basil
- Garlic
- Oregano
- Thyme
- Rosemary
- Sage

✓ **VINEGAR**
- Non-distilled Apple Cider
- Balsamic
- Cooking wine

✓ **STAPLES**
- Quinoa
- Wild rice
- Sesame seeds
- Capers
- Mustard (coarse-ground)
- Black, Green & Kalamata Olives
- Sundried Tomatoes
- Frozen shrimp
- Chicken sausages
- Veggie Burgers

Butter is Better

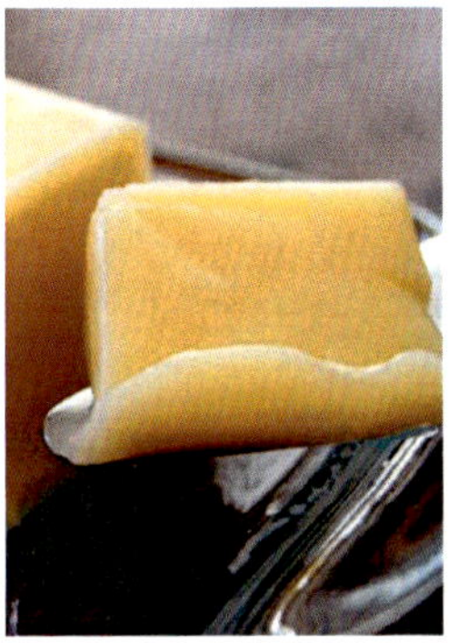

Margarine and shortening were the rage until evidence showed that hydrogenated oils and trans fats have had devastating effects on your health. Although trans fats in foods have been reduced, replacements, such as "inter-esterified" fats will prove even worse. The fact is that fake fats cannot be recognized or used by your body for anything constructive!

Margarine is made from vegetable oils, heated to extremely high temperatures. A nickel catalyst is added, along with hydrogen, to make it solid. Nickel is a toxic heavy metal and some amount always remains in the finished product. Because the heat turns oils rancid, deodorants are added to margarine to cover the smell. Finally, added colorings change margarine's unappetizing grey color to make it look like butter. You can't fool your body, though!

WHAT'S BETTER ABOUT BUTTER?

- **VITAMINS:** Butter contains vitamins, A, D, E, and K.
- **MINERALS:** Butter contains trace minerals, especially selenium, a powerful antioxidant (more than whole wheat or garlic); and supplies iodine, needed by the thyroid gland.
- **GOOD FATS:** About 15% of the fatty acids in butter are NOT stored as fat in the body, but are used by vital organs for energy. Butter contains *butyric acid*, a known anti-carcinogen, used for energy by the colon. *Lauric acid* is a potent antimicrobial and antifungal substance. *Conjugated linoleic acid* (CLA) also gives excellent protection against cancer.

BE SURE TO BUY ORGANIC!

Source: Stephen Byrnes, ND, RNCP, from mercola.com

BEWARE OF THE SUGAR MONSTER!

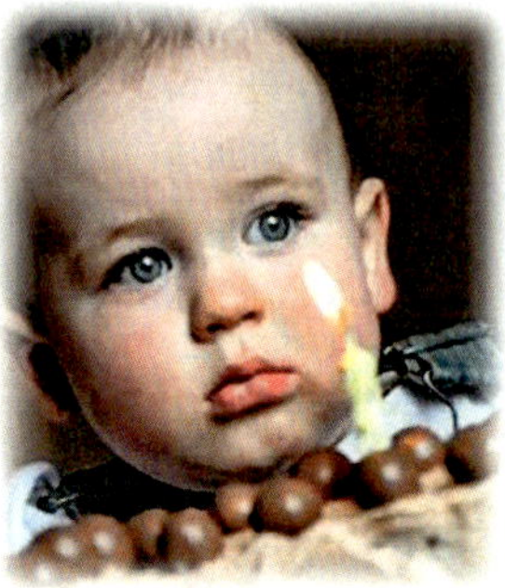

The poor kid never stood a chance. When Matthew's parents invited us to his first birthday party, he seemed somewhat over-whelmed, sitting in his high chair, surrounded by his family and their friends. He looked mystified by the singing and fiery candle atop the birthday cake. When his mom put a piece with icing in front of him, Matthew grasped the cake in one hand, then both hands, squeezing the icing between his chubby little fingers. One hand went to his mouth and, as soon as the sugary icing touched his tongue, his face screwed up in a scowl.

Matthew sat as if stunned, while his one-year-old brain went on a frenzied and futile search for a frame of reference in memory, and was forced to create a new one.

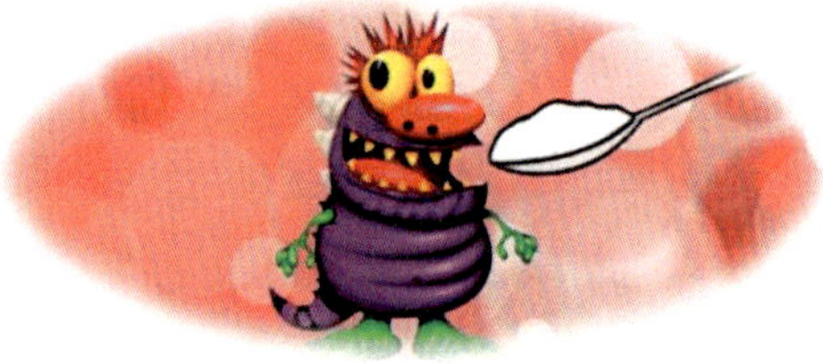

With a spoonful of icing, Matthew's mom encouraged a second bite. Matthew reached out eagerly, eyes wide, and plunged his mouth onto the spoon.

We were witnessing, in the space of less than 5 minutes, the birth of an addiction that threatened to run, and later ruin, Matthew's life.

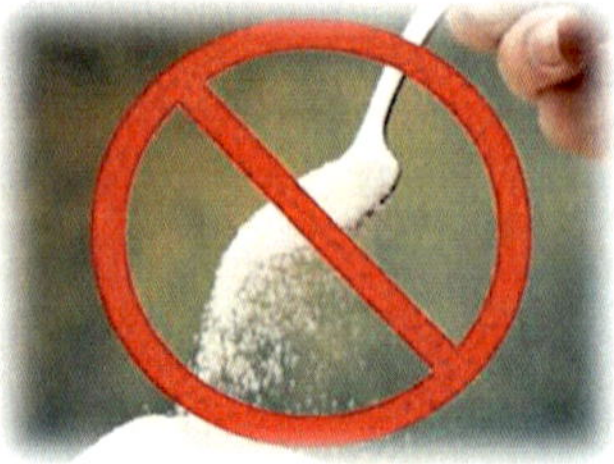

Sugar, in the form of glucose, is the fuel your cells convert into energy from foods you eat and liquids you drink. Glucose is absorbed from digesting *whole foods* and is released relatively slowly into the blood stream.

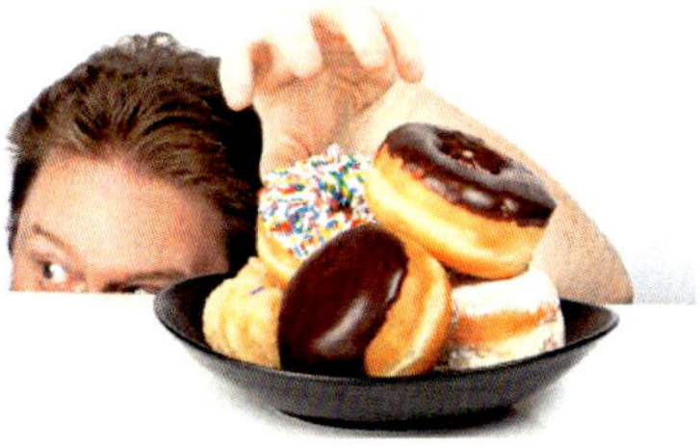

Refined sugars break down fast. For example, sucrose and high-fructose corn syrup (HFCS) in processed foods, fast food, "junk food," juices, and sodas, flood the blood stream with sugar, requiring huge amounts of insulin to be produced. The ultimate result of repeated, long term sugar overconsumption is chronic, degenerative disease, including insulin resistance and diabetes, and a host of unpleasant and unnecessary side effects.

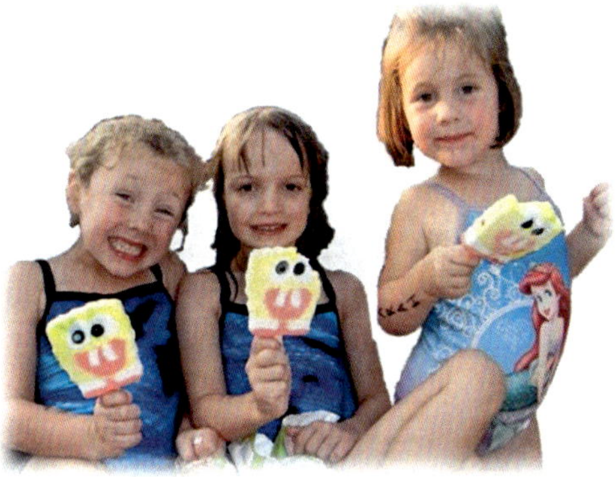

Refined sugar contains no protein, vitamins, fiber, minerals, or antioxidants; indeed, it seems to deplete these nutrients. Add its stimulant properties, and, *"Sugar is an addictive drug,"* says Dr. Christiane Northrup, a leading authority in the field of women's health and wellness. Dr. Robert Lustig, a specialist on pediatric hormone disorders and the leading expert in childhood obesity at the University of California, San Francisco School of Medicine, is one of many experts who argue that sugar – white or brown, from beets or cane, and high-fructose corn syrup (HFCS) – is a "toxin," or a "poison."

Artificial Sweeteners Are Even Worse!

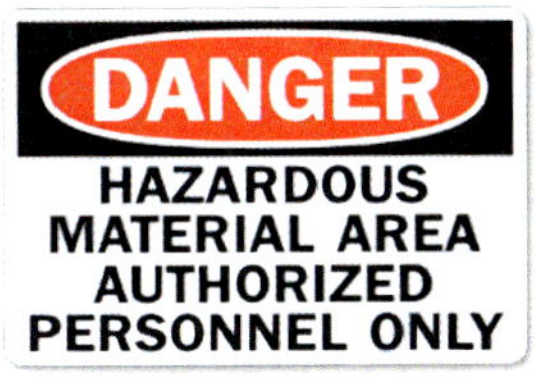

No matter which man-made sweetener you name – Aspartame (Equal® and others), Sucralose (Splenda®), Saccharin (Sweet'N Low®) – they all have *seriously* toxic effects. If a product is labeled "Diet" or "Sugar-Free," leave it on the shelf!

So...What Can You Use?

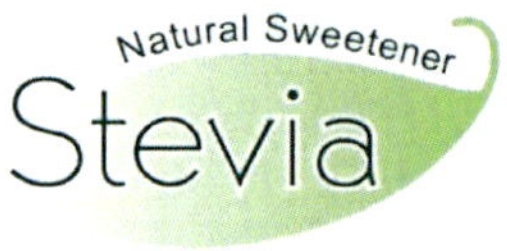

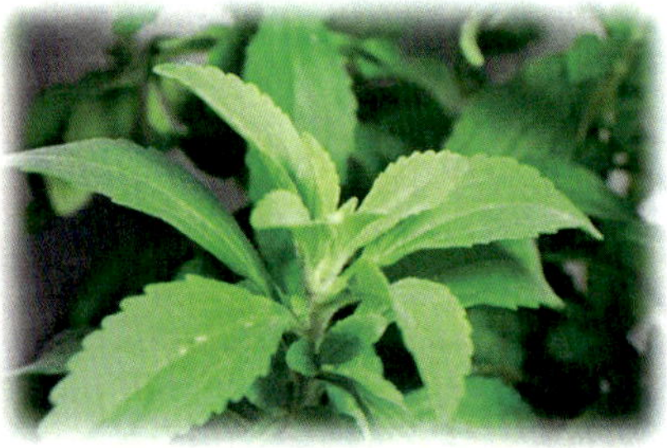

STEVIA is an herb, the extract of which is many times sweeter than sugar. In its pure form *(not combined with any other substances as are some products, such as Truvia®)*, **STEVIA** has no known toxicity, does not affect blood sugar levels or harm the liver. Its taste can be bitter if too much is used, so we prefer using liquid **STEVIA**, rather than powder, because the liquid is easier to measure consistently.

- **MONK FRUIT EXTRACT** is an all-natural sweetener that doesn't affect blood sugar. When mixed with other natural products to reduce its sweetness, it is easier to measure and use in cooking and baking.
- **DARK MAPLE SYRUP** is recommended for the **10-Day Lemonade Cleanse** because of the nutrients it contains, and to sweeten the lemonade; however, we *don't* recommend it for regular use.
- **HONEY** can be used *sparingly*, but make sure it's raw and locally harvested.
- **SUGAR ALCOHOLS** for sweetening include erythritol, xylitol, lactitol, and maltitol. All are touted as "natural sweeteners," but all of them must have fermenting agents added to manufacture them, and that makes us immediately suspicious. Of all the sugar alcohols listed, erythritol appears to be the least objectionable.

When you *must* have something sweet, get as close to nature as possible, and go easy.

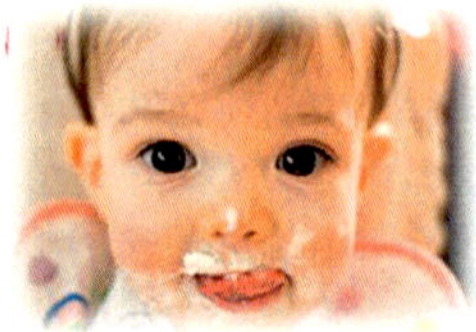

Microwaves Are For Cell Phones, Not Bodies!

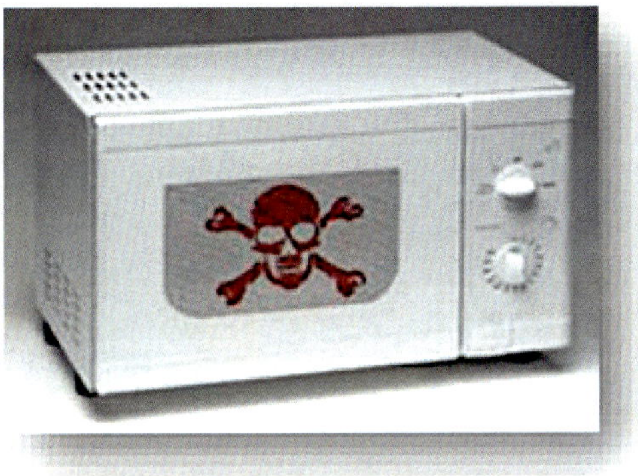

A quick internet search should convince any reasonable person to use a microwave oven only to heat something you don't intend to put in your mouth! Microwave ovens change the molecular structure of anything heated in them, and once you consume it, your blood changes too...and not for the better.

By all means do your own investigation, but while you're at it, consider this excerpt from page 43 of the book, *Comparative Study of Food Prepared Conventionally and in the Microwave Oven* (Raum & Zelt, 1992), by Doctors Hans Hertel and Bernard Blanc:

"A basic hypothesis of natural medicine states that the introduction into the human body of molecules and energies, to which it is not accustomed, is much more likely to cause harm than good.

"Microwaved food contains both molecules and energies not present in food cooked in the way humans have been cooking food since the discovery of fire. Microwave energy from the sun and other stars is *direct* current based. Artificially produced microwaves, including those in ovens, are produced from *alternating* current and force a billion or more polarity reversals per second in every food molecule they hit.

"The production of unnatural molecules is inevitable. Naturally occurring amino acids have been observed to undergo changes in shape, and transformation into toxic forms, under the impact of microwaves produced in ovens.

"One short-term study found significant and disturbing

changes in the blood of individuals consuming microwaved milk and vegetables. Eight volunteers consumed various combinations of the same foods cooked different ways.

"All foods processed through microwave ovens caused changes in the blood of the volunteers. Hemoglobin levels decreased and white cell levels and cholesterol levels increased over all."

A 6th Grader's science project was to water plants with regular water and water that had been microwaved. Her project and pictures have been circulated throughout the internet for years. As you look at the pictures below, imagine what happens inside your own body!

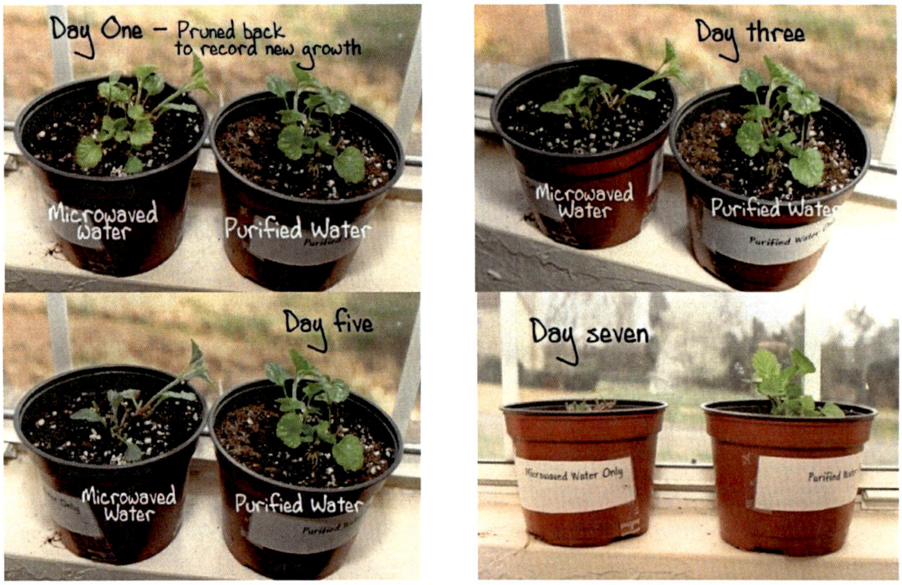

Find a health care professional whose office performs live blood cell analysis and do your own experiment to see for yourself the difference that microwaved foods and beverages make in the quality of your own blood.

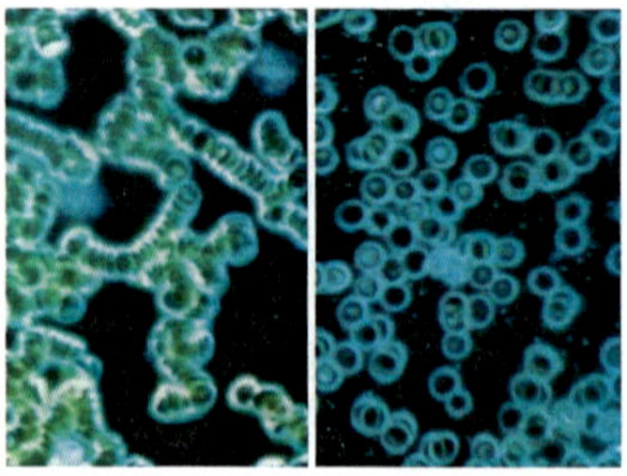

Which is the normal blood here?

TAP, TAP, TAP ... LEARN "EFT"

Millions of people worldwide have been helped by a simple tapping technique, called EFT (*Emotional Freedom Technique*). It's a tapping procedure based on a series of acupuncture meridian points, combined with concentration on a condition or other issue you want to heal. Literally hundreds of conditions have been helped by EFT: allergies, weight loss, post-traumatic stress disorder (PTSD), bed-wetting, asthma, chronic back pain, to name only a few.

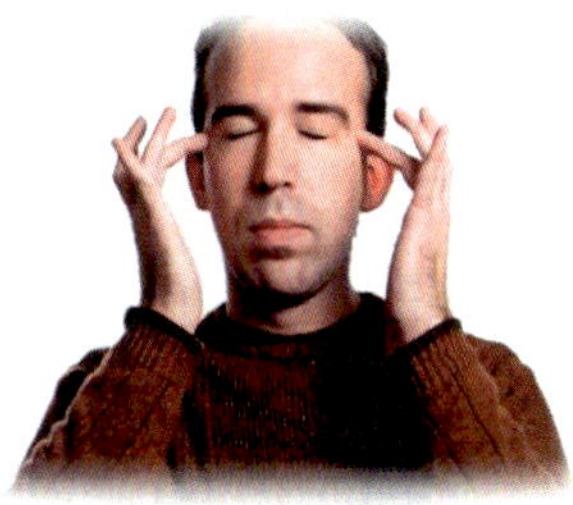

A simplified version of EFT is illustrated below:

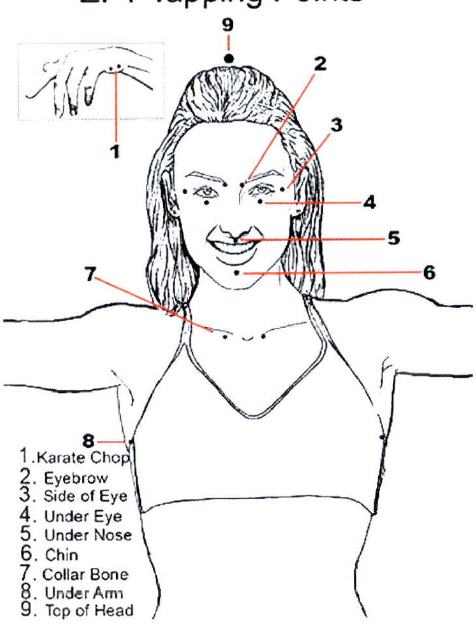

1. Rate the severity of the condition you want better on a 0-10 scale.
2. Use 2 finger tips, tap firmly with a drumming motion on each pressure point.
3. On the first point, tap while inserting the condition or problem to be solved into this sentence: "*Even though I have this ______, I deeply and completely accept myself.*" Repeat this 3 times.
4. Tap around the remaining points once, repeating "*this (problem)*," throughout the sequence of points.
5. At the end, rate the severity again and repeat the steps above until the severity is "0," altering the statements as needed to notice improvement.

For more information and resources on EFT, go to www.TheTappingSolution.com

Lots More How To's and Other Treasures

When you visit *CleansingRoadmap.com*

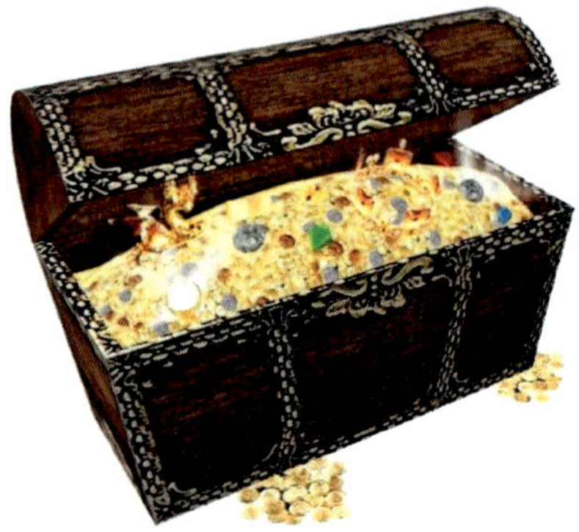

- **VIDEOS** – Access 20 videos answering the most important questions about Nutritional Cleansing and bonus videos which ensure your success. We've done the work. Just watch and follow along!
- **CHEAT SHEETS** – for **Belly Breathing**, the **Victory March**, our fast and delicious breakfast shake recipe, pH testing checklist, and more!
- **ACTION GUIDES** – Let us walk you through the steps that lead to success, whether it's losing weight, getting through caffeine withdrawal, or getting the most from your cleanses!
- **RESOURCES AND BEST SOURCES** – Find out what's worth watching and who's worth tracking! If you want to take your precious time searching through mountains of information and countless web sites, trying to find the stuff you need and the information you seek, be our guest, but chances are, we've already found most of what you'll need.
- **RECOMMENDED READING** – When it comes to health and wellness, authorities abound and very few agree. The good news is that the list is fairly short and the authors we trust get results. Have an authority you'd like us to check out? Let us know. We'll tell you what we think!

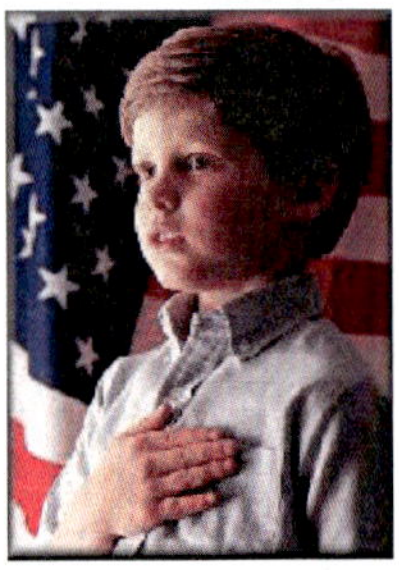

HERE'S OUR PLEDGE: We will *ONLY* share what passes the "100% test" we defined on Page 3. When anything is found to create more stress than benefit, we won't waste your time.

"...let your word be 'Yes, Yes,' or 'No, No.'"

(Matthew 5:37, NASB)

INDEX

You are now equipped to fly over, through, and past all limitations, and live in total freedom!

Get lots of extra content FREE at
www.WholeLifeWholeHealth.com

Add Your Own Resources and Notes

Get lots of extra content FREE at

www.WholeLifeWholeHealth.com

Divine Health
is Your Original Design